PSYCHOANALYSIS, THE BODY, AND THE OEDIPAL PLOT

Psychoanalysis, the Body, and the Oedipal Plot is a new radical departure in psychoanalytic exposition. An attempt is made to convey, in a language accessible for people from different disciplines, some of the most difficult processes that conform our subjectivity and our concept of difference and alterity.

Containing both significant theoretical material and applications of the theory to clinical psychoanalytic practice, this book offers the latest thinking on the importance of the body in psychoanalytic theory. *Psychoanalysis, the Body, and the Oedipal Plot* will be of interest to psychoanalysts, philosophers, and cultural theorists.

Fernanda Magallanes is a psychoanalyst and associate professor in the department of Philosophy at the Universidad Iberoamericana, Mexico City. She works at the intersection between psychoanalysis, feminism, and theories of corporeality.

PSYCHOANALYSIS, THE BODY, AND THE OEDIPAL PLOT

A Critical Re-Imaging of the Body in Psychoanalysis

Fernanda Magallanes

Routledge
Taylor & Francis Group
LONDON AND NEW YORK

First published 2019
by Routledge
2 Park Square, Milton Park, Abingdon, Oxon OX14 4RN

and by Routledge
52 Vanderbilt Avenue, New York, NY 10017

Routledge is an imprint of the Taylor & Francis Group, an informa business

British Library Cataloguing in Publication Data
A catalogue record for this book is available from the British Library

Library of Congress Cataloging-in-Publication Data
A catalog record for this book has been requested

ISBN: 978-1-138-38842-0 (hbk)
ISBN: 978-1-138-39126-0 (pbk)
ISBN: 978-0-429-42281-2 (ebk)

Typeset in Bembo
by Taylor & Francis Books

CONTENTS

ACKNOWLEDGEMENTS

I want to thank Judith Butler for her insightful feedback, her patience and attentive reading of this manuscript. I have been honored by her generosity in sharing her thoughts and her encouragement of mine. I also offer my appreciation, admiration and gratitude to Paul B. Preciado, Patricia Gherovici, Rosaura Martínez, Alfredo Valencia and Griselda Sánchez. They have transformed their geniality into a gift by assuming the compromise of thinking of the world despite its horrors. I feel very fortunate to have been able to receive what they share in different forms, and this book is here to present what their gift has particularly inspired in my thinking.

Thanks to Rachel West who has worked with me on the edition of this project since January 2017. Her hosting of my words helped transform them into a more readable text. Thanks to Alejandro Magallanes who designed the fantastic image for the cover of this book.

INTRODUCTION

Psychoanalysis, the Body and the Oedipal Plot is a new departure in psychoanalytic exposition. It begins with an attempt to convey in language accessible to people from different disciplines, some of the most difficult processes that conform our subjectivity and our concept of difference and alterity. This book proposes a reformulation of how we think of the body, bodily formation, the image of the body and its relation to emplotments and alterity. I also dismantle the Oedipal Complex as a central concept of psychoanalytic theory by critically thinking of the Oedipal Scenario as an epochal emplotment of the body that reproduces patriarchy. In this text, the body and the Oedipal are not only thought of within the psychoanalytic domain but also they are also restated to bring an ethical formulation of non-violence to our current cultural domain.

This book sums up my ideas on an array of concepts that captured my interest while thoroughly studying psychoanalytic theory. These ideas were shaped and transformed during my 10 short years of clinical experience, supervision and teaching, and the adventure of 14 years as an analysand on two different couches. Although some parts of this book may appear to be pure metapsychology, certain strong experiences my body underwent in psychoanalysis were the inspiration for this theoretical endeavor, without which it would never have been written. These experiences have had a transformative effect and have encouraged me to relate to others in new ways. They also inspired a critical reading of Freud's work, and although my reading sometimes pushes against classic Freudian theory, it never ceases to use that theory as a departure for thinking of ways that may alleviate social and psychic suffering.

This revision of Freudian theory will begin with a review of some of the fundamental concepts in psychoanalysis. In psychoanalytic theory, psychic and physical development of the human infant is enabled by its relationship to its progenitors. This relationship is configured through the encounter of their bodies. Although the term body has been thought of in many ways, the concept of body I use in this book is taken from Paul B. Preciado's Testo Junkie, where he defined the body as a sensorial-cultural archive that contains images, narratives, and daily cultural practices. This body is a somatic-psychic unity.

Using the lense of this definition, Part I presents a revision of the concept of the body in Freud's complete works. It also discusses the work of Jean Laplanche, Esther Bick, Françoise Dolto, Piera Aulagnier, Joyce McDougall and Richard Wollheim to explore further the image of the body, the body-ego and the primary forms in which difference is inscribed. Part I revises these metapsychological writings to explain the process by which images and representations hold the body. It proposes that how a body is represented determines the form in which abjection is produced and shows how the image of the body can become fractured and broken. Also discussed is how the meanings and significance that we attach to our materiality to become bodies as archives do not float free of that materiality. The fundamental tenet that to become a body we necessarily ascribe to emplotments that allow us to belong to culture is critically depicted. This revision facilitates a reformulation of corporeality in psychoanalytic theory.

Part I introduces the idea that bodies are subject to historical change and therefore to different emplotments in time. This part explores the concept of the body-ego and the image of the body to theorize about the linkages and breakages among body images and how these links organize in an emplotment. Part I also discusses how through symptoms bodies manifest the very quality of what is difficult to represent. Inspired by Preciado's Somatheque, I address how bodies can also manifest what he called epistemic crisis. An epistemic crisis of the body refers to a consequence of abrupt changes in the set of images and narratives that configure what a body is. Adding this perspective to psychoanalytic theory, I became particularly interested in the transmission of images and narratives that form the body. I explain that to psychoanalysis it is the caregiver that transmits culture and that which is transmitted forms the limits of the body, but culture is subject to change through iterability and therefore what is transmitted configures different kinds of bodies. These new bodies challenge the previous limits of culture and an epistemic crisis ensues. Such was the case of bodies in Freud's time who faced the fall of the Pater Familias and is the case of bodies today who manifest another kind of fall because of the rise of capitalism, the current political situation of the world and technological advances.

Part II explores how the concept of the body becomes even more intricate when we consider the Oedipal Complex, a term used by Freud to describe the universal trend of humans to desire parricide and incest. Freud placed the prohibitions of parricide and incest as central to the formation of the body because it explained the symptoms of the bodies of his time. Freud's theories use the Oedipal Plot to give an approximation of how a body forms and how it is limited and structured. When using this term, I refer to the universalizing storyline that Freud created with his appropriation of the tragedy of *Oedipus Rex*. This storyline has generated misunderstanding because of its insistence that all unconscious material be interpreted through the Oedipal Scene. In Freudian theory, this is the only plot that organizes the body symbolically. Part II makes an argument for a revision of the Oedipal Complex. It gives an account of how under this plot, bodies have formed their images to belong to the existing androcratic order in culture, but other plots that symbolically organize the body may exist for those bodies that are outside that patriarchal order. In this sense, this book is also a feminist deconstruction as it finds a way to dislocate Oedipus as the exclusive emplotment of the body. Freud's Oedipal Plot constituted a discourse on a way of being a body within a specific family configuration and influenced the current expectations of what is considered to be normal. But as is frequently observed in psychoanalytic practice, bodies today manifest different symptoms and psychic mechanisms than the bodies Freud observed in his day.

The fact that the symptoms of today are different from the clinical manifestations documented in Freud's time is forcing analysts to consider different interpretations. The most popular thesis has been that the Oedipal Plot does not represent the clinical manifestations of today's bodies, and that contemporary symptoms have either a narcissistic or pre-oedipal genesis. Part II discusses the resistance analysts have to thinking of other emplotments. It also critiques the specific way that Oedipus has been thought of in psychoanalytic theory and how its use as the only available emplotment has had a certain agency over bodies that inflict violence as it makes many bodies abject. Part II proposes that as psychoanalysts we work with the iterability of the sign of Oedipus and focus on Oedipus at Colonus as a supplement to Freud's reading of *Oedipus Rex*. It discusses other possibilities for the sign of Oedipus within the psychoanalytic domain and explores the potential consequences that this shift could have on the status of unrepresentability that many of today's bodies manifest. The shift of focus to Oedipus in Colonus allows Derrida's concept of hospitality to be inserted into the Oedipal sign and this opens up the possibility to relate to difference and otherness in a way that does not resolve into abjection. My theory has ethical implications for clinical practice and social phenomena and also aspires to be a contribution to other disciplines.

I ask that as you read this work, you undertake the intimate emprise of imagining how the discussed concepts could apply to your concerns. Towards the end of the book, I present concrete examples of plots that exceed the Oedipal, examples that I hope will illustrate the importance of my theory. I also discuss some advances in technology that, by changing the limits and capabilities of today's bodies, are making the mandate of a single binary and patriarchal emplotment obsolete. This book aims to show the profound effect rethinking the Oedipal could have on psychoanalytic listening. Instead of being complicit in the violence of abjection, if psychoanalysts open a symbolic space for alterity, it may contribute to a decrease in all forms of violence. I am sure that as pure metapsychology, *Psychoanalysis, the Body and the Oedipal Plot* has different applications that I did not think of. It would give me great pleasure if you as readers take this theory to your particular contexts and help me to break, transform and deconstruct it.

PART I

Body formation in psychoanalysis

1

PRELIMINARY REMARKS ON THE BODY IN PSYCHOANALYSIS

To address the iterated problem of having a body, it is first necessary to elaborate the concept of the body used in psychoanalytic theory and the process by which this concept has been formed. Indubitably, the emergence of the body as a representation that is different from the biological body is a difficult subject, one that has been treated obscurely in the past. Psychoanalysts hold very different points of view about this concept. A neuropsychoanalytic approach to the body would be incompatible with the concept of body employed in this text. A body in psychoanalysis is not equivalent to a biological body. Although the term has been thought of in many ways, in this book, I used Paul Preciado's definition of the body in his conference Somatheque (2012). In this conference he stated that the body is a sensorial-cultural archive containing images, narratives, and daily cultural practices; it is a somatic-psychic unity. This idea differs from previous definitions of bodies considered as merely the physical structure and material substance of an individual.

The body is explained through Freud's work in terms of a sensorial-cultural archive: a surface of cultural inscription, an erogenous extension, a psychic apparatus, a mystic writing pad, a device that reproduces fiction, a scene of writing. He first wrote about this idea in his *Project for a Scientific Psychology* (1895), where he described the infant's primal hallucination or hallucination of the maternal breast.[1] The young infant cries as the breast is taken away, and then in response to that absence, the infant begins to represent what is no longer available to him. That absence of sensorial stimuli is the first bodily restriction which then prompts the infant to hallucinate. Hallucination provides satisfaction when the breast is not present. The hungry infant evokes the image of the maternal breast and for a short time, can wait for the mother to return. The young infant's hallucinatory activity includes affects and ideas that reenact its previous bodily experiences.

This imaging defines thing-presentations that connect to sensation and affect and is the process by which the infant organizes the absent mother as a whole object.

As the mother becomes that whole object, a difference between what is inside and outside appears. In the process of realizing that there is a difference between an object and oneself, the representation of the body as a whole object is created. This process allows the infant to become a body that is separate from the world. This body is no longer just biological but is a body immersed in the culture that sustains it. It is the primary caregiver who transmits to the infant the experience of its body being something different than the world. This experience is first represented by the mother, through her desires and her way of being in the world. So, in psychoanalytic theory, it is the mother's restriction and absence and the resulting frustration and displeasure experienced by the infant that enable the infant to become a body immersed in culture. Therefore, it is by way of bodily sensations that culture is transmitted.

The concept of the body becomes even more intricate when we consider the Oedipal Complex.[2] In Freudian theory, it is not only the absence of the maternal breast and the frustration the infant experiences in its relation with the primary caregiver which establish the limits of the body, but also the re-edition of the primitive relationship that occurs via the Oedipal Complex. In the caregiver-infant relationship, the infant's omnipotence is interdicted by the absence of the mother or caregiver, whereas in the Oedipal Complex, this proscription is due to the mother desiring something other than the infant. In *From the History of an Infantile Neurosis* (1918), Freud named the infant's vision of its mother desiring something other than itself; the Primal Scene. It is in this scene that the infant constitutes a subjective image of its body in relation to its parents. The infant assumes the interaction between its parents as a prohibition of incest (of not being the only thing the mother desires) and as a prohibition of killing the father (of killing that which the mother desires more than the infant). How a body forms and how it is limited and structured depends on the position that the infant takes regarding this scene.

Freud had the brilliant idea to listen to the bodies of his patients and conceived of a plot for those bodies using a Greek tragedy as the central image instead of thinking of their bodies as machines. He chose the Oedipal Complex that placed the prohibitions of parricide and incest as central to the formation of the body because it explained the symptoms of the bodies of his time. Freud's sensibility led him to perceive symptoms as expressions of the agonies of a plot. This way of listening to bodies is very relevant in the history of thought because bodies experience the agonies of their time and bodies express those agonies through symptoms.

The Oedipal Plot reveals how infants become bodies in culture through the assimilation of certain prohibitions that set in motion mechanisms by which their bodies find its limitations. The bodies of mothers or caregivers are imprinted by culture; they then transmit that culture, imprinting it in the bodies of those in their care. However, the only prohibitions circumscribed by Freud are those of incest and parricide. He thought of incest and parricide not only as representations within the body as an archive but also as an architectural matrix that contours the perceptual and cultural limitations of that body.

As it is frequently observed in psychoanalytic practice, bodies today manifest different symptoms and psychic mechanisms than the bodies Freud observed in his day. The fact that symptoms today are different from the clinical manifestations documented in Freud's time has forced analysts to come up with different interpretations. The variance in their interpretations has made evident a lack of consensus regarding the concept of body in psychoanalysis and has been a problem for the psychoanalytic field. My assertion is that many of us in this field have a resistance to write about the concept. This resistance points to a difficulty in assuming today's epistemic crisis, and therefore we are challenged to understand the manifestations of somatic-psychic pain encountered in our practice. The body as an archive changes in time as images, narratives and cultural practices change. The idea of what a body is and what sexual difference means determine the legitimacy of a body in society. Those ideas are transforming, and bodies that appear to be different to a heteropatriarchal society are relegated as those operating outside the limits of legitimacy.

In separate approaches, authors Élisabeth Roudinesco and Paul B. Preciado posit that some of the body manifestations seen today announce a plot that does not correspond to the Oedipal Plot. In *Inappropriate Bodies* (2014), Preciado states that today we are seeing a new epistemic crisis of the body, and proposes a study of the genealogy of power implicit to the body. He also points to the need to create new myths concerning the body. In *Por qué el Psicoanálisis se debe renovar?* by *El País* (2015), Roudinesco says that the Oedipal Complex must be removed, and a new myth should be used to understand bodies and sexual difference today. She mentions that some contemporary analysts have argued that homo-parental families do not correspond to the Oedipal Plot. Combining the statements of both authors would imply the following: some bodies are abject from the norm that the Oedipal Plot inflicts, so the plot should be replaced to ensure the representability of those bodies.

However, my assertion is that Oedipus as a sign has already been thought of in a specific way within psychoanalytic theory, and the linguistic sign of Oedipus has already had a certain agency over bodies in the cultural realm. Therefore, dismantling the Oedipal Plot and the implications it has had would require more than just eradicating the concept or substituting it with another myth. As I mentioned previously, today's bodies have been configured through this plot. So, if we are aware that the Oedipal Plot has been the agent that acts upon bodies, the abrupt substitution of this myth is not possible, as bodies have already been formed by it. Thus, even if today we were to replace the Oedipal myth with another myth, it would not change the effects that Oedipus as a linguistic sign has had on bodies. I think that the best use of the reiteration of Oedipus in psychoanalytic theory would not be to substitute another myth for Oedipus but to rethink Oedipus beyond the Oedipal Plot. Therefore, my proposal is supplementary to that of Preciado and Roudinesco, and that is to work with the iterability of Oedipus as a sign. Working with Oedipus in Sophocles could expand the range of themes that the Oedipal Plot offers for bodily formation, but doing so will require clarity regarding the concept of body being used and also that we recognize how the Oedipal Plot's continued operation in our cultural realm is making some bodies abject.

In *Bodies that Matter* (1993), Judith Butler refers to abject bodies as those that become bodies through an exclusionary matrix where they become relegated. She poses that these bodies form part of an illegible domain of those where they do not enjoy the status of being a body and live under the sign of the unlivable. The unintelligibility of these bodies circumscribes the intelligibility of others. Taking into account Butler's perspective on abjection in the cultural domain, I explore how abjection is sometimes reproduced within psychoanalysis as well. I contend that when the analyst describes a body as abject or unintelligible, in part they are doing so to maintain their identity as a psychoanalyst. Their interpretation of others as unintelligible reinforces their own intelligibility. This rigidity present in the illusory identity of the analyst bound to a specific interpretation of the sign of Oedipus may be interfering with our ability to understand other bodies. Alternative ways to listen have been proposed in psychoanalysis, but we still need to work more with the linguistic reiteration of Oedipus as a sign. I assert that it is irresponsible for an analyst to say that there are subjects that are impossible to analyze. Their inability to think outside of the confines of the Oedipal Plot makes bodies that don't correspond to it abject.

To continue to theorize on the relation between the body and the Oedipal Plot, it is necessary to delve further into what a body is in psychoanalysis and how this body forms. The writings of Sigmund Freud, Françoise Dolto, Piera Aulagnier and Jean Laplanche are among the most representative of the process of subjectivation as a process of embodiment within psychoanalysis. These authors agree that the body cannot be reduced to its biological status. The following chapters in Part I present a critical reading of their works on this subject and is the starting point to reformulate how bodily formation, the image of the body and their relation to emplotments and alterity are thought of.

Notes

1 The term *maternal breast* refers to any object that enables the infant's desire to feed or satisfy its physical needs. The term *mother* refers to the infant's first caregiver, through which desire is transmitted to the infant irrespective of that person's gender.

2 *Oedipal Complex* is a term used by Freud to describe the universal trend of humans to desire parricide and incest. It is a complex in the sense that Freud considered it to be an organized system that describes universal traits.

2

HYSTERIA

The agonies of an epistemic crisis of the body

This chapter will commence by exploring how a new concept of body emerged in the modern era. It was the study of hysteria that initiated a discussion about the definition of a body. This observation of hysterical patients marked the starting point for theorizing about the body and has traditionally been referred to as the beginning of psychoanalysis. The hysterical symptoms were what prompted in Jean-Martin Charcot and his students, including Freud, the necessary curiosity to rethink the concept of body, and then to write about it. Therefore, I will begin by giving an overview of this subject.

Much has been written about hysteria, as it is a millenary concept that has become polysemic in time. However, if we attempt to define hysteria, problems immediately arise as it is a word with a life of its own, one that escapes signification. Hysteria as a signifier has appeared distinctly over time, with different names and diverse symptoms. Sometimes it is conceived of as pathology, other times as a structure of personality, a simulation or a trick. In popular discourse, it is used to imply hyper-expressivity, ambivalence, theatricality and high emotion. According to Capellá (1996), hysteria has been seen through the lens of alternative paradigms of thought, including the supernatural/magic model and the scientific/rationalistic model. The second of these paradigms, the scientific/rationalistic model, sees this body from the perspective of an ostensibly superior reason that finds it pathognomonic. However, there is something about this manifestation that was not entirely captured by any of these paradigms, something that would explain why the symptoms seen in hysterical subjects are distinct in different eras. It is as though some bodies express what the world has not yet come to terms with. If psychiatric medicine only treats the symptoms of these patients, it fails to listen to what these bodies have to say. Jean-Martin Charcot founded the school of neurology in Paris at *L'Hôpital de la Salpêtrière*. The school was an acclaimed research center and teaching hospital where the recent advent of photography had been incorporated.

Creating photographic records was highly encouraged at the school as an adjunct to the study of pathology. Hysterical women were the most photographed population of patients within the hospital. These photographs produced a visual record of bodies that are paralyzed, scattered, unstable, in a state of dreaming, unpredictable, contorted, whimsical, enigmatic, slippery, not apprehensible, difficult to explain. Bodies with symptoms beyond a biological explanation, erogenous and invaded by constraining looks: bodies exposed to the avid gaze of the doctors who were supposed to know what had befallen the patient, but ironically, it was the bodies of the hysterical subjects that were the carrier of such knowledge.

Charcot's disciples studied hysteria thoroughly, and they described the phases of hysterical crisis as auras, an epileptic period, a period of grand movements, a phase of passional attitudes and terminal delirium. The pseudo-epileptic crises were given the name Charcotian crisis as though attempting to contain these bodies within the name of the master. Charcot later expounded that hysteria is caused by a physical trauma that gives place to symptoms only when there was psychic longing for the trauma to be processed. Doctors at *L'Hôpital Pitié de la Salpêtrière* in Paris were convinced that trophic disorders could be cured by hypnotic suggestion, so hypnosis was the technique most prevalently used on these patients by Charcot and his disciples.

The elaboration of theory concerning hysteria began by exploring its relation to the body. Pierre Janet theorized that hysteria is mainly a dissociation of a double consciousness. For him, a synthetic force formed by reason, reality and culture integrates the body, but that integrating force is reduced in hysteria. This reduction of consciousness leads to the emergence of those psychic forms he called "inferior" such as hyperemotionality, the instinctive and the demonic. These states were considered inferior, as they were associated with animal behavior.

During the same period that Freud studied hysteria, he was also describing and analyzing the laws of the psyche. His first theoretical approach on the subject was in his text *On the Psychical Mechanism of Hysterical Phenomena* (1893) where he stated a clear difference between a psychic body and a biological body (that from now on we will call soma to distinguish between the two). When explaining hysteria, Freud distanced himself from Charcot's discourse and stated that hysterical paralyzes are not caused by trauma, not even by a dynamic injury. Instead of attributing a physical origin to the manifestations of the body he proposed a psychic one (originating from a world of representations). He posed that hysterical symptoms such as paralysis are caused when one representation is excluded from the ego because of an overload of affect. It is as if one state of the body (consciousness) remains unaware of the other state (unconscious).

According to Postel and Quetel (1983) Freud and Janet questioned how a part of the body could be paralyzed, in the absence of an organic disease that would explain the paralysis. They suspected that what was actually at the root of hysteria was the concept of the body held at that time. Thus, it was the symptoms of those who had been confined as hysterical subjects that introduced important questions about the body and initiated the formulation of the concept of the body in psychoanalysis. The bodies of these subjects struggled to communicate their difficulty to find a place in the modern world. These women were not conscious of the message their body was manifesting; they merely suffered the symptoms of the epistemic crisis of the body of that era. The unconscious discontents of civilization were acting through them. Induction into civilization necessarily entails that others imprint culture in us. Because of this, bodies as archives are never complete, and we are open to what the unconscious says through us.

In *Inappropriate Bodies*, Preciado (2014) stated that the body of women as a reproductive space is a political fiction specific to the modern era. Before the 18th century, the uterus was represented as a floating base in a vacuous space that belonged to the Pater Familias. Reproduction was thought to take place in the drop of sperm and not within the body, and the resulting infant was considered a product of men and God. So ontologically speaking a woman's body was regarded as a failure. The belief that the Word of God sustained women's uteri fell to immanence as God fell[1] and the idea of the uterus belonging to women emerged. After the fall of this modern fiction, some women found it difficult to appropriate their own bodies; it was this struggle that appeared symptomatically in hysterical bodies. Their symptoms were manifestations of an epistemic crisis of the body. Hysteria was announcing a new era for the concept of the body: a body with a flying uterus that could not yet be appropriated but that was no longer in the space of the Pater Familias.

It is frequently said that hysterical subjects are revolutionary in the sense that their bodies speak of a truth that is invisible to the consciousness of society. It is important to clarify here that it is not the subjects themselves that are revolutionary, but the return of the unconscious, which is acting through them. They are not consciously offering up their bodies to make a statement, but are seized by a discourse that speaks through their bodies but which to them is incomprehensible.

Their body communicates what had been repressed and is not yet ready to be spoken. This reemergence of the repressed occurs when representations that had been too difficult for the subject to bear consciously return from repression. The very insistence of their symptoms now begs for the truth to be spoken.

Just as the hysterical subjects felt threatened by the content of what they repressed, the doctors at *L'Hôpital de la Salpêtrière* feared the symbolic content of their symptoms. Taking pictures of these women served as a defense, seeing them through a photographic gaze allowed the doctors to maintain a certain distance and avoid their fear of this encounter. Thanks to the wonderful book *Invention of Hysteria* by Didi-Hubermann (2004) we can see the rescued images of hysterical bodies and how they were distributed, studied, supervised and kept under control. Archives of written and photographic representations of mental illness soon transformed the Hysteria corridor of the Hospital into an iconographic landmark. So historically, the elaboration of the body schema in psychoanalysis began by working through the fears elicited by an unknown body that challenged the medical schema, a body whose defensive power was captured in the photographic gaze.

When Freud first formulated his general theory of psychology, his theorizing about the body repeated the approach used by the medical profession, a machinery of power that breaks down, catagorizes, pathologizes and objectifies the body.

However, to me, by questioning this strictly medical vision of the body Freud went beyond the medical discourse and his own identity as a doctor. His investigation led him to think of the broken, fractured, ruptured aspects of the body as openings through which the repressed returned. In his article *The Unconscious* (1915), Freud suggested that the unconscious exists precisely because the body is broken and never complete as a conscious and autonomous entity. What distinguished Freud's approach to hysteria was that instead of replicating the photographic gaze of his contemporaries, he attuned his ear to listen to what these bodies had to say. This specific listening of Freud's that listened to the symbolic content of their symptoms opened up the possibility for these subjects to talk about the root of their symptoms instead of their bodies speaking for them.

Since its beginnings, the unconscious and its relation to the body have been central to psychoanalysis. In psychoanalysis what is efficient cause for determining behavior is not the materiality of the body but, rather, the representation that materiality attaches to it anaclitically.

Note

1 By fall of God I refer to how modern men in the late 1800's did not believe in a patriarchal system anymore, they wanted to dethrone it (the European empire). Modern thinkers were coming to terms with a symbolic instance that had failed. An example of this is Nietzsche's death of God.

3

GENERAL REMARKS ON THE CONCEPT OF THE BODY

In *Project for a Scientific Psychology* (1895) Freud prefigured what later would be constituted as Freudian thought. Before he wrote this text, Freud thought of the sexual in mechanical terms, but not yet as sexuality. At that time he held the idea of an accumulation of energy (that would later be named drive) inserted into a reflex arc dynamic. This accumulation of energy then constituted different pathologies. He classified sexuality as a need (*ananké*) that demanded a specific action, much as hunger is a need.

By the time Freud wrote Draft B (1893), he was questioning whether anxiety neurosis was a hereditary effect or whether it was begotten from a sexual order. He had observed that there are periodical moments of uneasiness in women related to psychic trauma and thought the cure would be through discharging sexual energy. In other words, at that time for Freud, the body was a biological-mechanical unit whose functioning depended on the accumulation and release of energy. He considered psychic workings to be merely economic processes.

It wasn't until 1894, in *Studies on Hysteria* that was written with Josef Breuer, that Freud made a first sketch of the functioning of the mental apparatus that would disrupt this biological-mechanical model. They hypothesized that hysteria indicates the occurrence of a traumatic event during childhood and that the affective charge of the event endures as a memory that is acting as a foreign body. In this text, Breuer and Freud proposed that a cure for hysteria could be achieved not only with hypnosis but also through catharsis by discharging the overload of affect.

From this moment on, there was a significant problem for Freud in regards to his theoretical approach to the body. On the one hand, he was positing that the body is mechanical and works through loading and discharging. On the other, he was introducing the effects of memory into the scheme. Freud's understanding of a body as a machine that works by way of discharges of energy became more complex. His thoughts would later evolve into a psychoanalytic discourse when he grasped that the event produces traumatic effects in the body when it is remembered. For psychoanalysis, the body is a somatic-psychic archive of memories that communicates by way of symptoms; this body is not equivalent to the anatomic body.

In *Draft G* (1894), Freud drew a diagram, a scheme of the sexual, to theorize about melancholia and anesthesia. The draft seeks to show how a sexual object that appears (*Gegenstand*) travels to a terminal organ as a sensation at which point a reflex action occurs. The appearance of that sexual object stimulates the senses of the infant, by cathecting a group of traces. This process is what enables the infant to represent. Freud called this first representation of the *Gegenstand* an *objekt*. For this process to happen, a quantity of workforce (Freud called this Q) becomes a drive only when it takes on the function of representing. The drive does not belong to a physical body, it is intermediate between soma and psyche and gives rise to the psychic. It is a corporeal inner pressure that leads to an action of discharge, a continuity, force, movement, stream, an intense yearning, an aspiration that pushes, tightens and exerts effort. Script G introduced something of utmost importance to psychoanalysis: an object that appears to us (*Gegenstand*) is not the same as a represented object (*Objekt*). Also, the Q force or an instinct (which is merely organic) is not the same as a drive (which is an intermediate form of psychic life).

According to the Freudian concept of body, there is a clear distinction between instinct (*Instinkt*) and drive (*Trieb*), and this must be elucidated. In his reading of Freud, Laplanche maintained that both terms should be treated as equal. This confusion was due to errors in the translation of Freud's complete works, and it introduced a misconception related to the psychoanalytical theory of drives and the notion of animal instincts. The distinction that Freud makes between these two terms clarifies the difference between a body formed by representation and the materiality of the body. It was precisely this originality of thinking that led him to conceive of the unconscious and a body that is more than its biological matter.

In Freud's theory, the fact that humans represent their materiality makes them different from animals whose bodies function solely through biological instincts. For Laplanche (1984) an instinct (*Instinkt*) is the classic scheme of hereditary behavior belonging to an animal species that develops in a temporal sequence. A drive (*Trieb*) is a dynamic process that compels an organism towards an aim. *Trieb* comes from the German root *Trieben*, which means to push; Freud's use of it underscores the irrepressible character of a force that continually pushes. *Trieb* does not appear in Freudian texts until 1905 in *The Three Essays on the Theory of Sexuality*. It is important to observe that the Freudian concept of drive arrived first in these three essays that describe human sexuality. Sexuality emerges as the representation of the sexual. The Freudian conception of drive dismantles the classical notion of instinct.

His idea of partial drives introduced the idea that in the beginning sexual drives exist in a polymorphic form and suppress tension. The term drive appeared for the first time in Freud's writings in 1905, before that, drives were understood in terms of the conflicting energy (*Reiz*) to which the organism is subjected. Later, in 1920, he named them as two opposite forces: the death drive and the drives of life. Drives of life represent the object, and the death drive unlinks one representation from another. In Freud's complete works, humans are always subjected to a force that represents the body and another force that unlinks representations and fragments the body. The energetic notion of the psychic apparatus began to be considered as more than an organic body, and other investigations of his contemporaries pointed towards a similar conclusion. In 1886, Freud argued that a defense (repression) was an unconscious mechanism that subsumes a representation charged with an affect that is difficult to bear as it is caused by the primary seduction of an other (caregiver). This primary seduction is re-edited in the different stages of development as the libidinal energy moves.

In *Screen Memories* (1899), Freud theorized about memory to elucidate the presence of amnesia in some of his hysterical subjects. Freud was questioning whether one could trust the memory of traumatic sexual events to be true. For a long time, Freud was a seeker of a kind of truth that used the model of an archeological excavation of a memory. He sought a truth that would correspond to what "really" happened. However, this hypothesis changed over time as it became evident to him that it is memory that mediates the access to reality. He began to theorize that life events are stored as traces. These traces retain the representations of the memory impressions that provoked an intense affect while other elements of the most decisive memories are forgotten. The way we forget is not by dismissing the memory from our mind, but by consigning it to obscurity. The representation is retained unconsciously as an omission.

Freud was intrigued by the subject of memory and seduction, in *Letter 69* to Fliess (1897), he wrote "And now I want to confide in you immediately the great secret that has been slowly dawning on me in the last few months. I no longer believe in my neurotics." He no longer believed that the seduction had happened literally and posed that the seductions his hysterical analysands spoke of were a phantasy of abuse.[1] To him, this phantasy of abuse is a distorted memory that seeks to re-edit something that had happened before (the primary seduction of the caregiver). Freud's understanding was that associations, as linked together in the analysand's discourse, correspond to a complex organization of memory. He compared memory to a system of archives that group representations together so that what one remembers is not necessarily the same as what actually happened. Then, although memories do not apprehend exactly what happened, there is still some veracity in them. Veracity is at the core of the body's fiction as phantasy and representation were initiated in pure material reality. This is how the idea of a psychic life enters the scene, one that is distinct from material reality.

According to Freud's thesis of phantasy, reality is only the product of the falsehood inherent to the act of representing. It is not that what the patients said is less real, but that reality is always mediated through phantasy. So, as the process of embodiment happens through representing, if superimposed representations give form to the body, then it is the ability to phantasize that allows an infant to become human. It could be inferred that for Freud, psychic reality is dependent upon somatic reality but, at the same time, never constrained by it. This overlapped body creates a new way of being a body, the body he had visualized in his studies on hysteria. It is the body of the caregiver with its memories, phantasy and history, which charges and gives life to a soma. The world of representation is mediated by phantasy because the infant is libidinized by a human who is already inserted in culture.

When Freud wrote *Three Essays on The Theory of Sexuality* (1905), he gave examples of the phantasies children have related to sexual difference and the purpose of sexuality. For him, sexuality implied a re-edition of the sexual, sexuality and the sexual being two different concepts. The sexual refers to the charging and discharging forces of the soma, whereas, sexuality relates to the representation of the sexual. Sexuality is present when representation exists beyond the basic needs of the biological body; when what is longed for is not a bodily necessity (hunger). Therefore, the human body needs others to intervene to satisfy what is beyond its biological needs. The body is incomplete as it is always longing for more, a reality that is not only circumscribed by its biology. Because of its inclination to represent, the body is destined to keep on morphing until the biological body is taken away by death. The death of the soma might be imagined as violent irruption that kills representation, phantasy, and memory.

In 1905, Freud inquired into the process by which the infant starts to represent images. He described the breast as the first object of satisfaction, one that affords the infant the opportunity to notice that there is something other than its corporeality. The infant experiences satisfaction when nursing and when the breast is absent, the infant represents the breast and starts to long for it as an object beyond the satisfaction of its hunger. The drive that was once directed towards the breast becomes autoerotic when the breast is lost. Through a hallucination of satisfaction, the absence of the breast is represented. This hallucination which is a product of autoerotism enables the infant to represent both its corporeality and an enigmatic world (the lost breast). Then, it is only because of the intervention of a caregiver that humans can assimilate their own existence and desire a satisfaction that exceeds the biological necessities (being fed).

Freud referred to the stage of personality development extending from about seven years of age to the beginning of puberty as the latency period. The primary relation between the infant and the caregiver re-edits after this latency period. The primary relation is retranslated a posteriori into a false memory by the condensation of images. Once again, Freud's theory of memory after the fact points to a body that fabricates itself in a belated understanding or retroactive attribution: a body of representation. Here rests the ultimate importance of listening in psychoanalysis. It is a method that is not about documenting the clinical history of facts that compose a person's life or past, but rather it is a way of listening to how a story has been registered, written and erased in the psychic body in a timeless present.

Capellá (1996), when commenting on Freud's concept of memory, stressed the importance of phantasy and explained that the fundamental factor in memory is not whether a person has many or few phantasies but how they are organized, that is, what underlies and organizes all the phantasies together as a fundamental phantasy. First, the phantasy is organized according to the vicissitudes of the drives, and then it is re-edited. A body, as we are now referring to it, is an archive that absorbs a set of cultural codes via its caregiver. It is a body that comes into existence by way of word-representation. The infant's psychic value emerges as a body that is capable of representing and therefore can phantasize using the language it has imbibed. Through phantasy, a psychic operation of a symbolic nature occurs and places the body in a position of subjectivity in relation to another body.

Previously, I mentioned how Freud's thinking about hysteria led him to conclude that a body attaches itself anaclitically to the soma and also inspired him to develop his first sketch of the process of subjectivation. Later on, in *The Ego and the Id*, Freud said that in the primitive oral state, it is impossible for the infant to differentiate between object investment and identification. He said that one could suppose that erotic aspirations are felt as needs because object investments come from the Id. In this text, Freud made a distinction between erotic aspirations and biological needs. Necessities are felt as erotic aspirations only in a moment a posteriori.

Mexican psychoanalyst Alfredo Valencia explained in his article *El Objeto del Psicoanálisis* (2017) that this is why the analyst thinks of the body in relation to the drives and their vicissitudes. To psychoanalysts, the body is erogenous, which is different to how neuroscientists, neurologists or cognitive psychologists think of the body. In psychoanalysis, the concept of drive is not a biological element of the body. The body is something that aspires, desires and is driven towards the object it longs for. In the function of representation that allows the soma to become a body, there is also a delay that is regulated by the pleasure principle. This delay is what allows the soma to avoid completely discharging itself and for the infant to start representing. The pleasure principle is frequently mentioned throughout Freud's texts but two of the most important texts where this concept appears are: *A Project for Scientific Psychology* (1885) and *Beyond the Pleasure Principle* (1920).

In these texts, he proposed that one of the principles that rule psychic activity is the pleasure principle, which seeks pleasure and to avoid displeasure. Displeasure means an increase in the energy of excitation while with pleasure there is a decrease. This means that to Freud, the soma's discharge of energy works in a mechanical way. Should there be total discharge, the soma would not have the energy it requires to sustain life. The pleasure principle also describes the capacity to defer gratification when circumstantial reality disallows its immediate gratification. Then, representing is an act of discharging energy with a delay. When obtainment of pleasure from the object per se is no longer available, then discharge occurs while creating an image of an object. If the infant were not immersed in the experience of becoming a body by way of representation, then its biological body would cry until there was a total discharge of energy. The pleasure principle serves as a barrier that protects the body from complete discharges of energy that could lead to death.

If there is no barrier to protect the body from total discharge, the body does not exist as different from another body. The delay given by the pleasure principle allows representation and therefore, representation of another person. Only by representation do we encounter the other, therefore any encounter between the body and the world is difficult. The relationship that the body establishes with the world is always mediated by what we suppose the other to be. Some analysts such as Donald Winnicott, Michael Balint and Otto Kernberg have split the concept of reality between internal and external, external reality being something different from the act of representing. This, however, goes against Freud's theory that says there is no such thing as a reality free of representation. For him, the experience of reality is only possible through a body that links representations and through the phantasy of what that reality is.

It is thanks to the deferral of gratification caused by the pleasure principle that the psychic apparatus works to inhibit the discharge of energy and to prevent an inscription of a perception (a trace) from being charged excessively. The pleasure principle prevents the trace from being immediately charged, so thing-representations do not appear as *Gegenstand* anymore when the infant evokes them. At that moment the infant experiences how perception does not create the pure materiality of things. It then starts to elaborate word representations, and this complex of unified traces creates a remembrance. This can happen because a limit has been established between the body and the other that is effective enough for the infant to understand that the *Gegenstand* is lost. If this process of representation through deferral of the discharge does not happen, the infant might in effect perceive partial objects that had been traced as real instead of evoking them with its mind through memory. Such failures of representation are frequently what is happening in psychosis, where for example a person might actually see the materiality of a gigantic hand talking to them. So then, when the inhibitory process works and representation occurs, the limits of the body are preserved. Therefore, we can say that the pleasure principle through its deferral of the discharge helps to prevent the body from losing its unity.

As the unity of the body is safeguarded, others are understood to be total objects. The infant is then able to choose new objects to represent other than the first object it encountered (caregiver). The possibility of an individual choosing one object over another depends on how much the representation of the object is similar but not equal to the first mnemic trace. Not only are the body and the world configured by the representations around that trace, but the identification process also occurs in that very same way. We choose the object we identify with by employing the model sketched in that first trace. As we look for what is new, we are longing for the object that was lost.

As has been established, Freud first conceived of the psychic apparatus as a machine that discharges. In the case of needs like hunger, the force of hunger acts incessantly on the biological body so no discharge can end the tension this produces. Change may occur for the infant only when the caregiver arrives with sustenance. The caregiver experiences displeasure when sensing the vulnerability of the child because memory triggers a complex of similarity. So they rescue its soma from this primary helplessness (*hilflosigkeit*), and by attending to the infant, the caregiver feels relief. The infant is rescued from its vulnerability by its caregiver, and by this process, its soma becomes humanized. In this sense, everybody's life is in debt to another.

When a similar other (caregiver) attends to the infant's needs, a memory trace is imprinted. At the same time, an experience of satisfaction occurs and cancels the internal stimulus. The thing that will satisfy the infant is an X, within the representation that is imprinted. The X is something unknown and unrepresentable. The caregiver will not consciously know what that X is and neither will the infant. I think that this X is what later on is called the unconscious in Freudian theory. Freud discussed this experience of satisfaction in *The Interpretation of Dreams*. He stated that the subject always looks for an object to satisfy its drives. However, no object will satisfy the subject. This longing for satisfaction comes from the relation to the original object. Desire is an attempt to reestablish the primary satisfaction with the first object that was lost. Based on this explanation, one would think that there is a sort of inherent desire in any subject, but there is no inherent desire as its origin is not merely biological. At first, the specific action of the caregiver satisfies the infant's hunger; then, the infant begins to demand to be fed. In the very process of making that demand, something else is added to that need than just the satisfaction of its bodily need. It is that added residue that becomes desire.

From then on, there is no complementarity between the subject and its object. No object fully satisfies us; complete satisfaction becomes only an aspiration. Therein resides the importance of the experience of satisfaction for the formation of a body that desires. After that first experience of satisfaction, a tension is not discharged, as no object fully satisfies the subject. The tension inherent in desiring prevails, and the simple act of desiring is pleasurable. Desire is never fully satisfied as it is always looking for new objects to represent the lost *Gegenstand*. It is only by way of this process of appearance and disappearance that a body that desires is constituted and the soma is humanized.

In conclusion, there are two births: delivery from the womb and psychic birth. The body is structured through psychic birth, an event that can only happen if the mother is invested in the infant. Psychoanalysis is the only discipline that sees the infant, as the caregiver's phallus. The infant is so essential to the caregiver that it phantasmatically completes her and ties into her desire. As the newborn psyche (referring to the second birth) represents the lost object, achieving completeness proves to be impossible. The infant, from then on, is condemned to a process of re-signification due to the loss of the object. Whatever ¨*His majesty the baby*¨ lost is no longer what he is. This loss constitutes his passing from being an omnipotent body to having a body. The loss of the object allows the infant to signify the limits of its body. It is only because of this loss that the infant can be an agent in the construction of its own body. Everything in the psychic apparatus will work to desire that object that is lost. Therefore, representing causes the soma of the body to disappear. The more we continue to represent objects, the farther we get from being pure physicality. But, it is only by way of the physical body that the second body appears. To psychoanalysis, there is a foreign body that emerges in an intermediate space between the soma and culture. This body is a somatic-cultural archive, which keeps on representing and undoing itself. The performativity of the body depends on a dynamic of representing, remembering and forgetting.

Note

1 Regardless of whether the abuse was real or phantasy, the fact that it was mostly women not men who were reporting this abuse speaks of a misogynistic cultural reality that is encrypted in the representation of these memories.

4

FROM BEING A BODY TO HAVING A BODY

In Freudian theory, the body is not given in the beginning; one is not born with a body, but it is built by way of representation. As explained by Freud in *Project for a Scientific Psychology* (1895), a new psychical action is necessary for the constitution of the body; the introduction of the soma to language. As soon as language intervenes in the body and we are able to represent it, we live the experience of the body in terms of having a body, not only being one. To understand how we go from being a body to having one, we must first understand the Freudian notion of narcissism. Freud designated the stage in which a body is primarily constituted as narcissism. In *On Narcissism* (1914) he said that at the beginning of a human life there is no unity of the dispersed libido, it has to be developed. As the autoerotic drives are primordial, the child's autoerotism needs a new psychical action to take place for narcissism to be constituted; this action allows the ego and the body to unify the disperse libidinal forces.

In *Studies on Hysteria* (1893), Freud differentiated hysterical paralysis from organic paralysis and remarked that hysterical paralysis does not answer to a biological etiology, but to the return of unconscious word-representations. He addressed this topic of language as representation and elucidated how it influences the body in his text *The Unconscious* (1915). In this work Freud introduced the concept of organ-speech,[1] which is a characteristic symptom of schizophrenia. At the onset of schizophrenia, a series of linguistic alterations and references to organs and body innervations come to the fore. What happens to language in schizophrenia is that there is no articulation between a thing representation (unconscious level) and word-representation (preconscious level). The word-representations of the body break and words substitute things but do not represent them. The body speaks, but not in metaphors as in hysterical conversion. This break in word-representations means that psychotics cannot represent themselves in symbolic terms and are still the same body as the representation of their caregiver. Consequently, they do not have a body; they are a body.

Joyce McDougall also wrote about somatic and psychic bodies and she elaborated on how being a body is different from having a body. In *Plea for a Measure of Abnormality* (1993), McDougall theorized about the psychosomatic body and explained it as being two bodies (soma) in one head. By this, she was stating something similar to what Freud said about organ-speech. By two bodies in one head, McDougall meant that the psychosomatic body occurs when neither the mother nor the infant have been able to represent their body, and are unable to differentiate their bodies one from another. Also, she explained that displeasure enables a body to accumulate charges and those charges build a connection between the soma and the psyche. The process of representing is then a painful but necessary process to build connections between soma and psyche. This connection enables a person to ask for help when in pain. The line that distinguishes between physical and psychic pain is subtle and may be confusing as pain hides an inherent paradox where painful experiences may be confused with painful corporal sensations (somatic). That is why, for McDougall, the body (referring to the soma) has the status of an object of the psyche (referring to the body as representation).

The body to McDougall (1993) is a body of representation, as it is to Freud. She wrote that the feeling of identity rests on the certainty that one lives in one's own skin. To her, in neurosis, repressed phantasies of the erogenous body create symptoms. In the case of neurosis, symptoms are formed by the return of the repressed, but in psychosomatic functioning, the representations that are inserted in the body are not formed enough to be repressed. The soma is cathected, and its bodily manifestations only discharge energy but do not represent. McDougall used the expression "two bodies in one head," meaning that the caregiver or mother and the infant become one shared body. The somatic body has two instances in the same person. To her, it is as if these two deaf bodies in one head get charged but do not communicate through representing, creating an effect of two competing monologs. This break in communication happens when no word-representation divides the soma and transforms it into a body of representation.

In *Theaters of the Body* (1989), McDougall wrote that designating someone as a "neurotic," a "psychotic," a "pervert," or a "psychosomatic" is a form of name calling. It reduces the complexity of what a body is, and it is a method of exercising power over patients' bodies. To her, the complexity of a representational body speaks of different dramas and representations. The world is a stage of dramas just as the body is a drama in of itself. In the same text, McDougall said that everyone has conflicts and areas vulnerable to psychosomatic breakdown, psychosis or the creation of perverse phantasies. What she stated is important. The body as representation is always vulnerable to psychosomatic breakdown, one may have a body, but that body has places where it is broken, cracked, damaged, defective, fragmented, mutilated. In other words, the body is incomplete, its unity illusory.

McDougall (1989) continued by saying that bodies are constituted by a number of characters that are frequently operating in complete contradiction to one another, causing conflict and mental pain. The different characters are constantly seeking their particular aims on the stage that constitutes our individual bodies.

These psychic plays may be performed in the theater of our own minds (body); for example, free association immediately reveals how a body is constituted by many characters. These characters are also projected and unconsciously played out in other people's bodies or in institutions.

An integration of McDougall's ideas with my revision of Freud would be that others figured as characters live within a body as an archive of sensations and representation. Some of those characters may be expelled or projected from the body. The characters (objects) on the stage (body of representation) give an illusion of unity to the body. Elements that are expelled from the mind institute a break in the body, a space of rupture; this gap where representation does not occur threatens the body's illusion of integrity. As long as elements and characters become represented, they are not expelled from the body, and that gap does not appear. If this representation is effective, one has a body. Having a body is about representing images, being a body is when we are not able to represent enough to appropriate a body. We are constantly swayed by the interaction between those two ways of functioning, having and being a body.

Note

1 Freud explained the term organ speech by describing what happened to a woman undergoing psychoanalysis with Tausk. He explains that schizophrenics speak a meaningful language that is syntactically and morphologically similar to ordinary language, but is qualitatively different in terms of semantics and pragmatics. Words and sentences are not representational or symbolic. It is a language of equivalence, immediacy and action. He called this language "organ speech" as it makes no distinction between body and world.

5

THE BODY-EGO

Although there are few explicit references to the expression body-ego in Freud's writings, the underlining idea is recurrent in his complete works. For Freud, the body-ego was the organizing basis of the structure of the body. In *The Ego and the Id* (1923) he defined the body-ego as a psychic projection of the soma's surface. In this chapter, I will present a revision of this concept in his metapsychological writings to stress the importance that primary experiences play in the organization of a proto-symbolic way of being a body. I will also elaborate a deeper understanding of body-ego and address more specifically how this organization enables the body to appear as a body archive that represents images.

As a body is immersed in language, it becomes of primary importance for an analyst to listen to the resonance that appears in his or her own body when an analysand speaks; also, for the analyst to observe how their words act in the patient's body, for example when the analysand cries, has a sudden urge to get up, go to the restroom, eat in the session, have coffee, light a cigarette or any other bodily action occurring during the session. Some common incidents are changes of voice, silences, sudden laughing or getting dizzy; other more rare reactions include hitting the analyst, shouting, vomiting or cutting themselves. According to McDougall (1989) by observing these bodily reactions, the analyst can see the mechanisms by which that patient's body was formed. I believe it is absolutely crucial that the analyst pays attention not only to the analysand's body reactions but also to his own. While free association opens a door to the world of representations of the subject, bodily reactions speak of how that language was constituted in the formation of a subject with a body.

I have stated that the infant's soma reacts to the body of the mother. Then, if an analysand reacts to an interpretation, the reaction may not be purely somatic but already a reaction that is pushing towards representation. We might then say that before the ego exists, there is a bodily ego that works towards the formation of the body as an archive (ego). Sometimes bodily reactions speak of symbolic content where the body is speaking in metaphors; such is the case with the symptoms of hysterical subjects described in Freud's *On the Psychical Mechanism of Hysterical Phenomena* (1893). Freud worked extensively with hysterical subjects to unmask the metaphoric content of their symptoms. However, sometimes in psychoanalytic sessions, analysands have bodily reactions that are not strictly related to symptoms, as their occurrence is not communicating a repressed content but are a direct discharge of the soma's energy. Whether they are symptoms or discharges, the analyst needs to listen to the mechanisms through which these bodily reactions appear during the session.

In Chapter 3, I explained how McDougall referred to psychosomatic functioning as two bodies in one head that get charged but do not communicate by way of representing, thus creating a dialogue between two deaf instances. In these cases, it is of primary importance that the analyst and the patient find a new representation of that body reaction. Not doing so would only reinforce the deafness of the psychic apparatus of the analysand. The analyst needs to listen to how the body is communicating and the mechanisms by which it works. It is very important to understand that bodily formation occurs first by way of a projection of the surface of the soma, the bodily ego.

I subscribe to the thesis of the body according to Freud, one that is constituted as representation, a body that is already broken in itself, divided between the represented and unrepresentable body, a division that proves to be the very condition of representation. French psychoanalyst Monique David-Ménard (1989) has argued that we tend to think of a developmental process that happens in a linear time. However, as I have explained, the process by which a soma becomes a body in culture is hypothetical as we can only give an account of the body through representation. The body is constantly being formed, so it cannot be said that there was one specific time when that representation happened, construction of a representational body is ongoing in a timeless present moment. By constantly representing itself, the body preserves its life and staves off the threat of dying. This threat exists because there is a space of unrepresentability where the death drive is active enough to unlink representation. So, there is a constant interaction between representing and undoing representation. If everything were represented, the body would be a closed entity where change would not occur. Unrepresentability is what allows the body to keep pushing towards representing. A constant interaction between representing and undoing representation happens. If everything were represented, the body would be a closed entity where change would not occur.

To further elaborate on how this process happens I will look at what Freud said about the bodily ego. In *The Ego and the Id* (1923), he stated:

> The ego is first and foremost a bodily ego; it is not merely a surface entity, but is itself the projection of a surface. If we wish to find an anatomical analogy for it we can best identify it with the 'cortical homunculus' of the anatomists, which stands on its head in the cortex, sticks up its heels, faces backward and, as we know, has its speech-area on the left-hand side. The ego is ultimately

> derived from bodily sensations, chiefly from those springing from the surface of the body. It may thus be regarded as a mental projection of the surface of the body, representing the superficies of the mental apparatus.

Therefore, it is the body-ego or bodily ego that is the nucleus of the ego. In Freud's complete works there is a distinction between the ego as the psychic apparatus, elaborated in *Project for a Scientific Psychology* (1895), and the ego as an instance or an agency within the psychic apparatus, depicted in *The Ego and the Id* (1923). The term Ich was used by Freud for both concepts. So, if we consider that the genesis of the ego is the genesis of the body, then the body emerges through the projection of the surface of the soma.

In his article *The Bodily Ego* (1982), Richard Wollheim expanded on Freud's thesis of the body-ego. He stated that the bodily ego might be related to the idea of identity. And, that if we speak of identity, we speak of the mechanisms of incorporation;[1] introjection of objects into the mind of the infant[2] and identification with those objects.[3] Then it is by introjection and incorporation that a body delimits itself. He questioned whether the mind and the soma are identical. To him, the idea of being a particular body corresponds to the soma's relation to objects in the world. Objects in the world are represented through the experience of somatic states (such as hunger). What is represented is not identical to somatic sensations in the sense that what is imprinted is not only the object of the world but the imprint in the soma that carries an "X" that is not representable. This unrepresentability, causes the infant to represent something that exceeds the somatic sensations, so it then tries to figure out what that object is. The concept may be clarified with the following example; the infant nurses from the breast, and after the breast is taken away, the infant replaces the satisfaction of breastfeeding with an image of the lost object (representation). But what the infant represents is not identical to the somatic sensations experienced by the infant. In other words, the infant hallucinates something other than its mother's milk.

Wollheim (1982) wondered whether self-representation and the object of phenomenology are distinct aspects of memory or whether self-representation is the derivative of the object that appears. Based on what has been discussed, it is a derivative relation, for according to Freud's *Draft G* (1894) there is a difference between *Gegenstand* – the object of phenomenology – and object – in the sense of self-representation. A self-representation emerges only after the *Gegenstand* is lost. Then, it could be said that the *Gegenstand* and object are not the same in the sense that the object that appears is never the same as what is represented. We may induce that to him what allows us to represent is the apparition of a consciousness of difference. The issue here is that the object that the infant represents is already something different from the infant's soma. The object of phenomenology is anaclitically attached to the object of representation. It is by virtue of the *Gegenstand*'s imprint in the biological body that representation occurs. The term anaclitical attachment does not imply that the object of phenomenology is lost forever. An anaclitical attachment means that the object of phenomenology is not completely lost because it left a trace and the representation (that inserts the possibility of difference) is attached to that trace. I want to stress that even if difference is needed for representation to occur, there is always a certain similarity between the represented object and the *Gegenstand*. Because what is represented originated in contact with the material world, then representation is always attached to reality (at least to some degree). This is why bodies serve as archives of unconscious cultural truths.

It is important to understand that the infant's first representations are anaclitically attached to reality, as introjection precedes the process of identification that occurs in the Oedipal Complex. To Wollheim (1982), beliefs are the ground that enables the process of introjection. When he used the word belief, he referred to a sensation that allows the infant to differentiate between what is good and bad for it. This concept of belief is equivalent to the Freudian concept of judgment of attribution stated in *Negation* (1925), which allows the infant's soma to choose certain representations over others and differentiate whether something is pleasurable or not. Wollheim (1982) called the process by which self-representation occurs, *make-believe*. He argued that the first imprint contains a belief that enables one representation to link with another. It is interesting to note that incorporation is a prototype for introjection[4] and identification. Incorporation refers to the mechanism by which the body represents a trace that contains a belief; thanks to the belief that is contained in the trace the infant can sense a notion of difference between it and the object. In this process, the infant introjects an object when the object has been sufficiently formed as a figure that is different from the infant. Introjection lays down a pattern for the process of identification to happen later. This identification contours the limits of the body through the prohibition of incest and parricide in the Oedipal Complex.

Wollheim (1982) posits that in the primary relationship with the caregiver, as representations become introjected, they may appear in one of two forms: as substantive or formal marks of internality. Substantive marks contour an object that the subject has in phantasy. A formal mark defines traits of character, imperviousness and reality testing which are ways of being. It could be said that Wollheim is thinking in terms of being a body and having one when he defines the marks that enable the representation of objects. This assertion that the marks of internality are what determine the difference between being and having a body gives continuity to the previous chapter in this book and reminds me of a quote of Freud's that continues to be very enigmatic. The quote is an attempt to explain the difference between being a body and having one. This note was found in Freud's drawer after his death and was published in *Findings, Ideas, Problems* (1938). It states:

> 'Having' and 'being' in children. Children like expressing an object-relation by an identification: 'I am the object.''Having' is the later of the two; after loss of the object it relapses into 'being.' Example: the breast. 'The breast is a part of me, I am the breast.' Only later: 'I have it'—that is, 'I am not it' …

By saying "I am the breast" the body is then the projection of a somatic surface represented by the idea of a breast. This is why I relocate Preciado's definition of the body as a sensorial-cultural archive into a reading of the Freudian Body. The body is a mental projection of the loss of the somatic surface, which first left a trace as a representation and later on is represented as a whole object. The process by which a body is configured is one of losing and recovering through representation that which was lost (the breast). In this quote, Freud is making a distinction between being an object, which is when there is no distinction between the infant's body and the caregiver's body, and having, where the infant is aware of a difference between itself and the breast. So then, the ability to represent implies an awareness of being different from the object. The infant's perception of difference may be a re-edition of a primal belief where the infant senses that the object is not identical to his soma.

Freud defined the first frustration as the absence of the breast experienced by the infant. This frustration allows it to become a body as it establishes the notion of difference. This first frustration transpires in the interaction between two bodies and is what allows the mechanism of introjection of an object to occur. The second frustration occurs with the Oedipal Complex and involves the interaction of three bodies. This Oedipal configuration is a re-edition of the first acknowledgment of difference. In the Complex, the understanding of difference is expanded to include the prohibition of incest and parricide, which mark the body as excluded from the relation of two parental figures where the infant is not the most important object. The Oedipal Plot appears in the cultural domain as a discourse that has been universalized. As a discourse, the Oedipal Plot enables us to represent the markers by which our bodies are constituted as an archive. But to me, becoming a body depends more on the establishment of difference enabled by belief and the mechanisms by which representation of the image of the body happen, than on the content of those representations. Those representations are subsumed to the Oedipal Plot, and therefore to representations of parricide and incest. In conclusion, what is most important to the central idea that is being developed in this work, is that to become a body we must represent a plot. Ideally, this plot would not only allow the body to be able to represent itself, but to represent difference from others and would foster the ability to value what is different in others. In the next chapter, I will continue to explore how a body represents itself and will discuss how language acts upon the body.

Notes

1 The idea of oral incorporation was first stated in *Totem and Taboo* where Freud defined it as a form of identification that has a somatic prototype that is cannibalistic: devouring, eating, ingesting, or keeping something inside oneself. This type of incorporation is frequent in melancholia where the subject identifies totally with objects that are lost.

2 Freud explained introjection as a mechanism of the instinct's relation to its object. Introjection is a primitive mechanism that has its somatic prototype in the act of incorporation. It implies the internalization of an entire relationship.

3 Freud defined the concept of identification as the process by which the subject finds similarities between himself and objects, characteristics of a person, ideals or partial objects. Identification always preserves the stamp of its earliest prototypes: incorporation and introjection.

4 Introjection of the object is the internalization of an entire relationship that comprehends more than a simple representation.

6

BICK, ANZIEU AND PIERA AULAGNIER

Both Esther Bick and Didier Anzieu put forward the thesis that the skin plays a primordial role in the formation of the Ego. In *The Experience of the Skin in Early Object Relations* (1968), Bick, using beautiful imagery, spoke of the body as a vulnerable state, one that may become unbound from its bodily source (the skin). She explained that the primary processes of bodily development are greatly influenced by the infant's dependence and separation from its caregiver. The most primitive parts of the personality are unconnected to each other; it is the infant's skin that contains them. For the skin to contain all parts of the personality, the infant must differentiate between what is internal and external. The mother's care and her response to the infant's dependency are what induce this awareness of difference. Dependency is crucial to reinforce the first skin in this period of fragility. If the caregiver's response is insufficient, the creation of an analogous double skin may occur to replace the integrity of the first one.

In *The Skin Ego* (1989) Didier Anzieu based his theory on the Freudian principle of the Body-Ego where bodily functions develop into mental states. To him, the development of the psychic apparatus is supported by successive ruptures that make it necessary for the organism to search for links between psychic functions and bodily functions. Anzieu also proposed that the skin surface of the body and the brain, are derivative of the same embryonic structure: the ectoderm. Following that logic, the skin is primordial as a provider of the constitutive representations and functions of the Ego. Anzieu thought that the drive toward attachment is of considerable importance to humans given that childhood lasts much longer than in other species. This drive is directed first towards the mother or caregiver and then extends to others. Contact, physical presence, sound images, cradling, availability for feeding, care and company, all provide the notion of an exterior reality and continuity. This prelinguistic communication provides a fundament for understanding languages.

Anzieu (1989) was more specific than Freud in explaining how the body is constituted through the body-ego; Freud stated the body-ego is built on organ sensation and Anzieu localized it in the skin. According to Anzieu, the ego is constituted from tactile experience. For him, a self exists before the ego as a body, as the self gives an account of the tactile experience, which becomes the ego. A primary prohibition takes effect that limits touching and a predominance of the visual substitutes that first tactile envelope. Representation then, comes first through the skin, after which it becomes visual and the representations associate preconsciously to form word representation. Expanding on this idea, he says that the skin-ego is intermediary between metaphor (thought as word representation) and concept (thought as visual representation).

According to Anzieu (1989), the ego encloses the psychic apparatus in the same way the skin encloses the body. He observed that some skin functions could be transposed onto the level of the skin-ego. These functions include; being able to contain thoughts, ideas and affects, provide a protective shield, register traces of primary communication with the outside world and manage inter-sensorial correspondence. Other skin functions that could be transposed are, to individuate, to support sexual excitation, and to recharge the libido. So in that sense, the skin-ego separates the inside from the outside of the body. The way Anzieu thought about the broken parts of the skin-ego is that they bear consequences for mental organization. He traced the body in visual arts, literature and painting and sometimes in psychodrama. This tracing was done from the perspective of an observer, not as an intervening analyst. As, for example, in the analysis he did of Francis Bacon's works. In Bacon's paintings, skin covers structures without bones. Anzieu interpreted these representations of boneless structures as extensions of an alcoholic ego where liquids were the only things contained.

In *The Ego and the Id* (1923) Freud maintained that the psychic apparatus (body) emerges from the organ (soma). Bick (1968) and Anzieu (1989) took this concept even further when they proposed that the psychic apparatus emerges specifically from the skin. For Anzieu, the sensorial experience in the skin then becomes visual. This model of thought raised a question, which went far beyond what Freud stated since for Freud it is the charges coming from the contact with another human that organize the unity of the body. Drives are the intermediaries for representation and serve to predispose the transformation of the soma into body. But for Anzieu, drives attach images so that representation occurs by way of a charge that moves from the skin to the eyes. Even if the theoretical approach is similar, something very different emerges. To Freud, the transformative effect depends on how the drive transforms the first trace into representation and for Anzieu; the superficies of the soma are what create representation. In Anzieu's perspective, there is already localized eroticism in the skin that travels to the eyes. Eroticism is created as a representation of the libidinal charges deposited in the soma. For Freud in *Three Essays on the Theory of Sexuality* (1905), representing a body starts with necessity (hunger), which is satisfied through the mouth. The absence of the object of satisfaction allows orality to become erogenous; this act of disappearance is what causes the body to represent. Freud's notion of drives offers a more complete account of how the bodily ego (soma) emerges into a body of representation. Drives then are the central concept in psychoanalysis, the pivot of metapsychology.

Anzieu's soma is even more passive than the Freudian soma. For Anzieu (1989) the skin is the bodily ego that is charged through contact with the other, it is as if none of the other organs are as important as the skin. Therefore, Freud's concept of reflexive action would only correspond to the skin. But when a baby cries, isn´t that body alternately inflated and deflated with air? How can one think of the initiation of erogenous charges as pertaining only to the skin? When a baby is born, a cry is what immediately emerges. One can see the inner part of the baby's body expanding and contracting. Then, considering that vulnerability of the baby: Why did Anzieu insist that the bodily ego is already localized in the skin as if the paramount need of the baby were to be embraced rather than to be fed? At least in this first stage, the important need for Freud is hunger. Of course, it is one thing to agree that every psychic function develops through a bodily function that is translated into a mental state. Anzieu's idea concerning the role of skin in the development of the body seems clear as well. To him, skin becomes erotically charged and in this way creates the world and the human body as a cultural somatic archive of representation. However, what some psychoanalysts continue to dispute is whether the skin is erotically charged at the same time as its basic physical needs are met, or only after they are satisfied.

The author Piera Aulagnier addressed the subject of the body-ego in *The Violence of Interpretation* (1975). Aulagnier highlighted the corporeal processes before the construction of the ego as a body as well as the failures that emerge in those processes that produce pathology, linguistic disturbances, and corporeal manifestations. For her, a representation and an instinctual representative are complementary. An instinctual representative is an idea or group of ideas that is cathected with a definite quota of libido. Aulagnier called the first sensorial experiences of the body pictographic representations. It is only later with the body's insertion into language that it can acknowledge the forces that operate in the space that surrounds it. For Aulagnier, the experiences that the infant has with language are responsible for an effect of redoubling of the psyche. From then on the body is split between the body and an agency that observes it. The psychic scaffolding organizes around that psychic agency as a place that is open and in constant exchange with the world around it.

When Aulagnier (1975) developed her thesis about how time intervenes in subjectivity, she identified three processes that unfold: original, primary and secondary. These modalities of psychic functioning are not present at the beginning of the infant's life but occur in linear temporality. She understood the original process as being the absence and presence of pleasure that leads to what she called "begetting." By that she meant that one's own activity of representation creates a pleasure state, engendering the object that causes that pleasure. The experience of the infant is that it is creating the maternal breast. Up until this point, what Aulagnier has said is a rephrasing of Freud's theory. However, she then goes on to elaborate on the theme, stating that the trace of this original process is *the pictogram.*

A pictogram is a prelinguistic seal, a painting, and a trace of an original encounter between the infant and an object. A *pictogram of fusion* is from the sphere of images and is a trace that provides the foundation for representation. It is the mother's function inscribed in the infant as a positive (+) charge that promotes an effect of linking and psychosomatic integration under the representation of Eros. By linking love and dependency, the mother establishes the measure for achieving pleasure. However, if displeasure prevails in the absence of the object a *pictogram of rejection* is represented. In a second moment, which Aulagnier equated to the primary process, phantasy is the representative activity that dominates. She defined it as a psychic activity characterized by the imaginary realization of desires to avoid the displeasure produced by the absence of the initial link to the mother. Aulagnier thought of the secondary process as a third moment, characterized by an idea-representation or enunciation. It is only when the infant enunciates that it can weave a past. The necessity to think, to question what one is thinking, having to create historic narrative for ourselves: that is the price we have to pay for the right to participate in culture.

To Aulagnier (1975), the figure of the mother becomes the spokeswoman of genealogy, the voice of enunciation. Hers is the voice that conveys the sociocultural discourse, the discourse of the parental couple and its families of origin. The sentences enunciated by the maternal voice are taken by the child to constitute a parental ego. The mother cathects the infant through the representations she weaves of her child. The caregiver weaves a libidinal plot that provides a psychic envelope that is necessary for the infant's becoming a body. Aulagnier spoke of a "shadow" that the object leaves in the infant's soma when the object is absent. A psychic body can't be created without a shadow that is represented and then spoken. The shadow may protect or be threatening, be benign or malignant, but it is always essential. Then for Aulagnier, it is the mother who cathects the body and creates the body of representation that does not correspond to anatomy that Freud wrote about.

Aulagnier went even further to claim that the mother's elections, thoughts, and discharges of pleasure are installed in the psyche of the child, and that the child is in a predicament as it is absolutely vulnerable and dependent on others. This process of installment is motivated by the mother's desire and although necessary and anticipatory, is quite violent. She called that act of investiture, primary violence. To say that subjectivity is in itself an act of violence is a strong statement to make. Aulagnier claimed that infants experience violence at its most exaggerated level because they lack freedom and autonomy to oppose the imposition that is implicit to the mother's care. If the primary violence surpasses its necessary character (inserting the infant into culture), it can become what Aulagnier called secondary violence. Secondary violence happens when the mother's cathexes in the child are too difficult to bear. In this case, the infant is psychically damaged and deprived of the right to think for itself. The child's incapacity to think autonomously forms a desire for immobility. With luck, the desire for immobility will revert in adolescence, a stage where relationships with new objects are conducive to breaking the paradigms of its infancy. Adolescence is not only a stage of hormonal and somatic changes but also a re-edition of previous object relations. In this stage, the psychic energy (libido) moves to different places in the body, and other objects become necessary to represent those physical changes. Piera Aulagnier stated that this re-edition is not linear but haphazard, serendipity, a situation where the new and what is different may appear and be linked to what has been lived previously; in other words, the body or ego is always mobilizing. For her, there is a memory fund, constituted in a primitive stage.

The memory fund keeps valuable experiences because of their affective intensity. As memories re-edit, the body can keep on historicizing about itself and the world. This principle work of memory and representation provides the infant with the capacity to understand difference and to engage with life. The two main functions of the body as representation are to guarantee identification and to create a phantasmatic capital. By phantasmatic capital, she meant a conjunction of representations that are kept in memory. Memories are a relational matrix, in the sense that psychic inscriptions recreate experiences with others. What constitutes memories as such is the mechanism of repression. It is the mechanism by which the unpleasurable is relinquished to the unconscious. Repression splits the subject into a conscious body and unknown forces. Unconscious forces are in constant dialogue with the conscious body in order to break with habitual thought and allow change to occur. Repression of the unconscious creates the possibility of a constant recreation of the body. As indicated earlier, a psychic redoubling occurs in the infant's psyche when it is exposed to language; this redoubling organizes around the spatial proportions of the soma. The body as an archive is open, in constant change and exchange with the world around it and in a continual dialogue with that which is unconscious.

It is decisive for my argument to begin thinking of the body as a place and the world as a projection of the body. I suggest that the thesis of the bodily ego leads us to posit that a body as an archive is created through the soma, and objects of the world are an extension of the body. Then, the body is a place, an archive that is the site or depository of cultural signifiers. The infant encrypts images of the world into its skin through the signifiers that the caregiver imparts. These signifiers carry a world that is culture and represented objects, and they are what transform the infant's soma into a body-place. So, it is the intrusion of these signifiers that saves the infant from primary vulnerability. This act is violent but also necessary for the infant to be inscribed as a body in the world.

This making of the body as a somatic-cultural archive is possible through a pictogram of fusion, which allows psychosomatic integration under the representation of Eros. But, if the experience of displeasure prevails over the experience of pleasure, problems in the integrity of the body-place arise. In *The Violence of Interpretation* (1975) Aulagnier said that the inability of the infant to inhabit its body is represented through a pictogram of rejection. To me, the idea of the pictogram of rejection speaks of abject bodies in society. The pictogram of rejection not only unlinks representations but delinks the body of the subject from its feeling of belonging to the world. Although there may be bodies that are absolutely inscribed by a pictogram of rejection and bodies that are absolutely inscribed through a pictogram of fusion, I think that in most cases, some bodies just get a bigger dose of one pictogram than the other. Piera Aulagnier work suggests that to be inscribed into the world as a life that matters, there must be a pictogram of fusion, as well as the capacity to represent images of oneself and the world and to keep on living. At the same time, however, a pictogram of rejection is inscribed, which creates the possibility of the irruption of a debonding force that unlinks the representations of the body.

If we combine Freud's ideas with Aulagnier's proposition, this debonding force may be understood as death driven because it unlinks representations and dismantles the illusion of integrity of the body-place. The pictogram of rejection enables a desire for immobility and acts upon the body making it abject. In this sense, abjection is a death-driven force that produces incapacity to think, to be critical and to be responsible towards others. As bodies, we are sometimes affected by a secondary violence that does not allow us to reason. Paradoxically, for an ethical relationship with others, we need to take responsibility for what the death drive unlinks, that which is unthinkable. Then, taking responsibility for alterity would require a better understanding of the death-driven force.

7

THE BODY AND THE DEATH DRIVE

The previous chapter discussed how drives are intermediary between the soma and the body, and how the soma and body are inseparable instances that transform each other. In the following chapter, the question will be developed of whether the transformations that the soma and the body effect on each other transform the paths of the death drive as well. To delve into this question and get a better idea of what unrepresentability in bodies means, I will review specific facets of Freud's theory of the death drive. Facets such as erogenous masochism and its relation to the death drive, repetition-compulsion as a derivative of the death drive, and the death drive's manifestation as guilt.

In *New Introductory Lectures* (1933), Freud referred to the drives as being mythical entities, magnificent in their indefiniteness, and said that the theory of the drives is the main mythology of humanity. If we go beyond the role the Oedipal myth plays in the constitution of humanity and think of the drives in this more ample context, we will have a more inclusive scheme with which to think of bodies, not only the Oedipal Plot. In *Instincts and their Vicissitudes* (1915) Freud defined the concept drive (*Trieb*) to be a concept on the frontier between the mental and the somatic, as the psychical representation of the stimuli originating from within the organism and reaching the mind. Although Freud located the source of the drive in the soma, he said that the drive is a concept in the frontier between the mental (body as an archive) and the somatic. The term *concept* may be confusing because a drive is not understood to be a word-representation, but a pre-representation in between the psychic and the somatic. We may consider Aulagnier's notion of the pictogram to be equivalent to the drive. It is a pre-representation with a force that pushes to represent (drives of life) or to unlink (death drive).

Freud presented his theory of drives in successive formulations. To make a clearer distinction when referring to the successive moments in the development of his theory of drives, I will speak of the different periods of formulation in his work. In his first formulation from 1905 to 1914, Freud recognized and counterposed sexual drives and self-preservation. Sexual drives are the energy that humans direct towards objects in the world and they tend to conserve the species. Self-preservation comprehends somatic reactions that allow one's own life to persist. The energy of those sexual drives is called libido while the energy of self-preservation is designated as interest. In *Three Essays on the theory of Sexuality* (1905) Freud insisted that in time sexual drives become independent from the death drive, but he did not explain how.

In *The Psycho-Analytic View of Psychogenic Disturbance of Vision* (1910) Freud claimed that all drives in the psyche either come from hunger or are striving for love. He also introduced the notion of ego drives and sexual drives. He conceptualized sexual drives as forces subsumed to the pleasure principle. The ego drives were those tending to self-preservation and serving as the agent of repression. He may have called them ego drives because they serve in the formation of the ego. He defined the concept of ego as both the subject and a set of representations that aim towards self-preservation. The difference between ego drives and sexual drives was not very clear in this text.

Ten years later, in *Beyond the Pleasure Principle* (1920), he introduced a fundamental category of the drives: the death drive. In this text, Freud no longer speaks of ego drives and now refers to the drives of life and the death drive as oppositional forces. The attachment between life and death drives results in aggression. If the death drive is attached to the drives of life, but the death drive prevails, that aggression is directed outwards as hostility and other destructive forces; whereas, if the exteriorization of the death drive is limited, aggression may be internalized and tends towards self-destruction. The attachment of these drives can also manifest in a sadistic form in what he called will to power or drive for power.

The death drive tends to reduce the energy of the soma, causing the living being to return to a state of unrepresentability. The destructiveness of the death drive does not support the conservation of the species. In *An Outline of Psycho-Analysis* (1938) Freud posed that in the psychic apparatus, there is an intrinsic conflict between self-preservation and preserving the life of the other. However, safeguarding our own life entails that we represent the objects of the world; therefore to live, we must protect others. This paradox shows that although at first abjection establishes the foundations of difference, our preservation requires that we transform our relation to difference. It is important that bodies struggle towards difference and also that they are open to others, even if that openness may at times be dangerous.

In *Beyond the Pleasure Principle* (1920), Freud expanded his idea that there is a pleasure principle that regulates mental functions. The ego as a body of representations works to seek pleasure through energetic equilibrium. The pleasure principle reigns in the mental apparatus, but there is a pleasure beyond that pleasure. That *beyond* is territory of the death drive, where the nirvana principle prevails. The nirvana principle tends to an absolute discharge of energy, a complete reduction of tension where difference and individuality are erased and annulled; where that which is alive, dies. Life may only subsist if the drives of life transform the nirvana principle into the pleasure principle. As the pleasure principle acts, energy is discharged with a delay. This delay also takes place because of the reality principle, which is the ability of the mind to assess the reality of the external world. The reality principle can be thought of as what allows the soma to create a bodily construction that is concordant with the soma and the world. It is of utmost importance to take a moment to observe what Freud is posing here. His theory suggests that by virtue of their representing function, the drives of life are not only intermediary between the soma and the body but are also transformative forces of the principles that regulate the psyche.

In *Beyond the Pleasure Principle* (1920), Freud continues to elaborate on the manifestations of the death drive. He posed that the main expression of the death drive is repetition-compulsion, understood as a phenomenon in which a person repeats events that happened to them previously or puts themselves in situations where that event will happen over and over again. He wrote that the death drive tends towards what is not different or new as it unlinks representations that would allow new possibilities to come into being, but in Freud's *Remembering, Repeating and Working-Through* (1914), we can see that he had come to understand repetition as a way of remembering. He posed that when the analyst is capable of transforming into words the patient's tendency to repeat certain actions, this awakens remembrance in the patient. He said that symbolization could only occur when repetition is subordinated to the pleasure principle, that is, a capacity to delay is needed to symbolize. Language is a form of symbolization that takes into account this delay. Therefore, Freud's example of the effect of the analyst converting the patient's tendency to repeat into words illustrates how the death drive may be transformed into life through the words of others.

Furthermore, others give life to the body of the subject not only in the first moments of life and the process of subjectivation but throughout their life. Following Freud's ideas in *Beyond the Pleasure Principle* (1920), repetition-compulsion acts as a counterforce to the pleasure principle, but paradoxically repetition instigates the creation of another kind of pleasure. He stated that repetition-compulsion is more original, more elemental, than the pleasure principle it dethrones. If the paths that the death drive takes are not in the direction of life, the concept of difference will not be understood. The death drive may only go in the direction of life if it is subsumed to the drives of life. The tendency towards life is a tendency that comprehends that we are different from others. Valuing difference is what prevents us from hate and destruction.

In *Instincts and their Vicissitudes* (1915), Freud described a relation between hate and the ego drives. To him, the prototypes of hate do not come from sexual life but from the ego's struggle for its conservation and affirmation. He wrote that in the process of subjectivation the origin of hate precedes that of love. So, we can say that the paths the drives take before the subject can love are full of vicissitudes. The death drive and drives of life continually link and unlink, they are in a constant dialogue that determines whether they create or destroy.

Before this, Freud considered that the pleasure principle worked because of the drives of life. But if repetition is understood as a derivative of the death drive and all drives repeat, we can assume that that which is relative to the drive is more directly related to the death drive than to the drives of life. Then the first or primary drive would be the death drive, and the drives of life would derive from their opposition to it, operating through the pleasure principle. The intrinsic and inevitable tendency of the soma is to live towards death. But in the process of bodily formation that takes place in the interaction of the infant and another, the pleasure principle acts so that life is also a procrastination that delays the realization of the death drive's aim towards death.

In *The Ego and the Id* (1923), Freud pointed to the silent functioning of the death drive; he wrote that the death drives are mute. Not only are the death drives mute (without manifestations) but they also push towards muteness when unlinking word-representations. In its purest form, the death drive is unrepresentability. Drives of life push towards representing and enable the body to speak. Freud found the manifestations of the drives of life easy to understand, but the concept of the death drive was more evasive, so he envisioned it as a drive of destruction in which hate prevails over love. This means that in its purest form, the death drive is unrepresentability acting over the body, in its mixed formed it has manifestations such as repetition, destruction, and aggression. However, if the drives of life give direction to the death drives in their attachment, the ability to make word-representations prevails. The drive of destruction links the drives of life and the death drive. The drives of life free the soma of the destructiveness of death drive by fusing with it.

The fusion of the drives follows two different paths. A part of the attachment of life and death is directed outwards to the external world, as aggression, while another portion is directed internally towards the organism. Life constitutes the act of representing while the death drive undoes representation. If life prevails, drives of life and the death drive will work towards cohesion, but if death prevails, the death drive will work to undo representation and will act unattached from the drives of life. In the relative equilibrium of the attachment of the death drive and the drives of life, a part of the death drive in its purest form takes a rest from representing, acting silently as it leads the organism on its inevitable path towards death. Referring to this issue, Freud maintained that every human being dies because of internal causes. The death drive is that internal force that seeks the organism's death.

In *Civilization and its Discontents* (1930) Freud wrote that guilt is another manifestation of the death drive and in *Analysis Terminable and Interminable* (1937) he went further to ascertain that a need to be punished emerges from something beyond the conflict between the ego and the superego. This issue is central to Freud's theory of guilt as it complements the thesis of guilt he established in *The Dissolution of the Oedipus Complex* (1924) and *Totem and Taboo* (1913) where guilt emerges after parricide or a phantasy of it has occurred. He stated that the punishment arising from guilt (masochistic) happens because the death drive unlinks energy from representation. Therefore, guilt occurs before the Oedipal Complex where Freud said that the superego forms. So the guilt inherent to the Oedipal Complex can be thought of as a re-edition of this more primary, masochistic guilt. Ergo, the Oedipal Plot may represent the very structure within which the drives work.

In *The Economic Problem of Masochism* (1924), erogenous masochism is defined as a form of satisfaction of the drives. Freud explained that when the death drive acts in the interior of the organism, primal sadism is indistinguishable from masochism. One force is directed towards objects while another force remains in the interior of the organism as a residue of erogenous masochism. This dynamic constitutes a basic dualism that later accounts for the ambivalence between love and hate in a subject's life. Then, this ambivalence can be understood in terms of how the drives work: hate has its origin in the ego's struggle to preserve and maintain itself; love for its part originates in the drives of life. This ambivalence between love and hate may explain why Freud gave so much importance to his interpretation that the Oedipal Plot was about the prohibition to kill (hate) and the prohibition of incest (love). I assert this because the limits of the body are formed by the re-edition of primal relationships in different stages of life. The subject's Oedipal ambivalence may be a way of representing the experience of the dualism of the drives.

The Economic Problem of Masochism (1924) explains that erogenous masochism is a residue of the death drive. Erogenous masochism emerges as a separate part of the soma and directs the libido elsewhere. It is through expelling erogenous masochism (making it abject) that the body as representation is created. Part of the death drive becomes separate from the part that is attached to the drives of life. This split of the death drive only happens if the body goes through the experience of a loss. In my assertion, as the breast is lost, the death drive in its pure form preserves itself by remaining separate from attachment. The body as an archive is created only by the linking of life and death, and it is undone when the death drive acts in its pure form. Then, if the body is that which struggles to represent, the death drive in its purest form is everything that is unrepresentable. Therefore, it is by virtue of what is unrepresentable or abject that we may represent our body. We need unrepresentability to have a body. Although what is unrepresentable constitutes the very condition for our existence, the task of life is to keep on representing that which is made abject and threatens us (death). It is precisely the act of representing that allows the body to assimilate difference beyond abjection.

Recapitulating a linear appreciation of how the soma becomes the body is a hypothetical task as to speak of the soma one is already inside of the sphere of representation. As theorizing is already the task of representing, we may think of the process in the following way: If a drive is a concept, a drive is either a pre-representation (pictogram) or a representation. The first, or one of the first representations, forms as the *Gegenstand* disappears. As it disappears, it starts to become an object by representing what was lost. The loss may only be represented because the imprint of that absence (X) gives rise to the drive as an intermediary status between soma and body. Therefore, the drive's origin is not only somatic but is also contained within this inscripted imprint (x). It is a concept but also a force, that pushes towards representation. As the object is lost, the concept (drive) is split into two main forms of drives: death drive and drives of life.

The first split is between death (unrepresentability) and life (representability). Drives of life sometimes act in their pure form and sometimes attach to the death drive to subsume it and represent what appeared before as unrepresentable. At the same time, the death drive in its pure form stays silent as it is not attached to the drives of life and contains everything that is unrepresentable; the expulsion of erogenous masochism is what enables this split. Erogenous masochism emerges when the libido is inwardly directed, and that happens through an automatic process that is not filtered by representation. The body continually creates itself by representing what appears as unrepresentable. It is this process that allows the unrepresentable to speak through us. Therefore, the split between what is representable and what is unrepresentable is what inaugurates the body as a cultural archive. The pleasure principle maintains a homeostasis of energetic charges that enables this split to be effective and the body archive to have narcissistic unity. This narcissistic unity configures the body as a body that is not only a material entity but also one of representation. To have the notion that my body is different from other bodies is already the result of the work of representing it. The split of the drives enables the body not only to have a narcissistic unity but also gives it the bases for the appreciation of difference.

The death drive in its pure form is necessarily abject from the body as an archive and does not belong to the somatic or psychic body but to a separate instance of unrepresentability. The subject is divided into a body that represents and an unrepresentable body. So seen in these terms, two instances exist: the body as an archive, and the unrepresentable or abject. Death is an unknown because it is abject. What is abject (by the act of the death drive in its purest form) and the body as an archive (where the death drive acts attached to the drives of life), positions the body as an archive in a dialectic relation to death. We have a body and keep on representing it towards death which is unrepresentable. Because of the division between the body as an archive and the unrepresentable, pure death is facing us all the time even if we are not aware of it.

If we understand the drive as a representation of the absence of an object, there is an inherent willingness to represent the unrepresentable place of absence. Death is absolute absence so representing is an important part of the struggle to prevent us from dying. We represent our bodies to struggle against the death drive in its pure form. If the death drive is subsumed to drives of life as we represent, the paths that the death drive takes may be transformed. If we do not continuously represent the body and the soma does not transform into something new, the path of the pure death drive acts with a greater force over the body as an archive. Then it can be said that new representations change the body as much as they transform the paths that the death drive takes by linking it to the drives of life.

The question that was crucial to Oedipus in Colonus was where he would be buried. Because the death drive had unlinked the representation of his body, he was now an abject figure. Oedipus' difficulty finding a place to die speaks of the status of unrepresentability of his body. As I have explained before, the world is the projection of the body, so, Oedipus' difficulty in finding a place to die may be speaking of the status of unrepresentability of his own body. By the time Oedipus' arrived in Colonus, he had already gouged his eyes out. His lack of a burial place, also speaks of the extent to which the death drive was influencing his body. So then being Oedipal does not only correspond to the Oedipal Complex of psychoanalytical theory where Oedipus gouges his eyes out as a punishment for committing incest and parricide. Body dismemberment and punishment may speak of something more than the guilt for transgressing these prohibitions. Françoise Dolto's hypothesis of the images of the body will elucidate how body images form and how they break so that we can further interpret the image of the body with a rereading of Oedipus' suffering.

8

FRANÇOISE DOLTO

The unconscious image and the function of language as a narcissistic bond

Françoise Dolto worked with children and observed the joy that children displayed when speaking about the drawings they made. She interpreted those drawings not as represented phantasy to decipher the structure of the unconscious but as a representation of the image of the bodies of the children. To Dolto (1984), the capacity of children to speak about their drawings re-edits the psychic instances of the subject. In other words, the children's image of the body is not the image of the drawings, but language creates the image of their body as they speak of it. To her, there is a saying encrypted in the body that waits to be deciphered. The image of the body is an image that waits to be spoken.

In *L'image inconsciente du corps* (1984) Dolto made a clear distinction between corporal scheme (soma) and image of the body (body as an archive). The corporal scheme provides a way for the body to live in contact with the physical world. The experience of what is real or not depends on the integrity of the soma and its muscle, bone or neurological injuries as much as of physiological sensations. Injuries in the biological organism may cause temporary or chronic disorders in the image of the body because of the interruption to parts of the body that are linked to language. That is, she took the soma to be the surface of the psychic body.

As an example of how language acts upon the body, I will now relate an urban legend from Mexico that I first heard from psychoanalyst Alfredo Valencia. The legend tells how a certain analyst who was very overweight had friends who would tease him about the size of his body. With considerable pride and good humor, he responded with the interpretation that they were envious that his somatic surface was bigger and therefore more generous in psychic pleasure than theirs. That analyst's capacity for bodily representation is fortunate, and the way he speaks of his corporal scheme shows he understands the meaning of difference beyond abjection. That is, when faced with the words of others, he assumed the signifier "large" as something that made him different from others. He did not answer by making himself abject or by making others abject but by giving them back a represented image of their bodies as envious bodies. With this example, I show how language transforms the body image and shows how linguistic performativity relies on the capacity to represent one's body. This also explains why integration of the changes made to the somatic form of the body such as organ transplantation, plastic surgery, or sex reassignment depend on how compatible these changes are with the subject's body image.

In *L'image inconsciente du corps* (1984) Dolto gives another example of this: when a corporal scheme altered by injury cohabits with an uninjured image of the body. After losing his legs, a child tells his mother how he will run and jump, but he is no longer able to do that. Talking with the subject about his illusions allows him to integrate the illusions regardless of the reality of his physical restrictions. To Dolto, this integration is symbolized by an image of the body. The evolution of the subject depends on the child's emotional relationship to its caregivers. This integration is possible if the child is loved and held and in an exchange of the creative resources of the caregiver, the image of the body structures is reformed.

The image of the body is connected to the subject and its history. It is eminently unconscious. It may turn preconscious when consciously associated with images of the body in the mimics of language and verbal language through metaphor and metonymy. This body image is the synthesis of emotional and inter-human experiences lived through the senses. A signifier is always attached to a somatic sensation.

The first symbolic incarnation of ourselves is the image of the body, and we desire whatever is a projection of this image. The object is desired to try to integrate that image. In other words we represent the world in order to have a body as an archive. To Dolto, previous to the conception of the infant, there is already unconscious desire in the mother. This desire influences the infant's body even before the infant can say "I." That is why Dolto says that the image of the body is an unconscious memory of an enigma.

The image of the body actualizes and changes through language, drawing, musical experiences, mimicry and gestures. According to Dolto, this image of the body is attached to the corporal scheme and is the support of narcissism. That is, the image of the body attaches to the corporal scheme. It is what Freud called the bodily ego and is the predecessor of the body as an archive as well. Dolto stated that the image of the body is a very fluid image since well before the formation of the ego.

To her, libido is in continual movement when relating to others. Libidinal movement may cause an archaic image of the body to return from the repressed. What Dolto said is the same as was reviewed in Freud's theory. The difference is that she stated very clearly that repressed elements are also images of the body. To her, desire is born from an immanent unconscious representation of the body. This unconscious she spoke of has certain representability. So as discussed in the previous chapter when speaking of death drives, we can say that the unconscious contains images of the body and other unrepresentable parts. For Freud, there is both the unconscious (X or the unrepresentable) and a dynamic unconscious (what is repressed).

In *An Outline of Psychoanalysis* (1938) Freud made clear that the death drive lacks representation and tends to unlink representations. It lacks residual representation and influences the subject to get rid of images. We may then assume that the death drive tends towards the destruction of representations of the body, which results in the destruction of the world as understood as a projection of the body. The death drive makes it impossible to represent some images of the body and the world because the world is an extension of the body.

For example, bodies that lack visibility in today's heteropatriarchal society are invisible because they are made abject by the society whose death drive posits them as unrepresentable. This death drive only sees bodies that identify with an image of a good citizen under patriarchal terms, and it makes women and other bodies it considers different abject. As we know, normality in these circumstances is not inclusive or kind. A good son of patriarchy in Ciudad Juárez may be a man who murders women. Women who are killed in Ciudad Juárez are not mentioned by name afterward; they are referred to as "las muertas de Juárez" (the dead women of Juarez) instead of naming them as individuals and explicitly saying that they were violently killed by men. An undetermined number of women have been murdered, and women continue to be killed every day. This form of patriarchy posits an X in those women as unrepresentable. It is not that the materiality of those women's bodies is not representable, but it is made unrepresentable by brutal misogyny that promotes unrepresentability even after destroying the materiality of those women's bodies.

When the death drive governs the drives of life, the death drive manifests itself as aggression and femicide. But the purest form of the death drive is that which insists on disappearance and unrepresentability: "las muertas." Although the number of women that have been murdered is horrifying, very few people participate in the marches to protest their deaths. The status of unrepresentability of these women makes it difficult to represent them. In terms of the death drive, that is even more deadly than killing them, which is already terrible. As bodies, sometimes we are afraid to see that bodies that are killed are also images of ourselves. Representing these bodies means legitimizing them as individuals. Naming the dead women and acknowledging that they were killed would give visibility to these bodies. Furthermore, if the bodies of these women had been represented by society instead of having been made abject, it could have prevented their being killed by men's aggression. This form of patriarchy validates the existence of men by making women abject. Later on, this example will help us understand how the Oedipal Plot invisibilizes some bodies and restricts the body from representing itself in a new way. By delimiting what can be represented, the Oedipal Plot has had an effect of limiting the appearance and acceptance of difference.

In *L'image inconsciente du corps* (1984) Dolto understood difference as a concept that is inscribed in the infant from a constant re-edition of the image of the body and the introjection of difference between the infant and the caregiver. The interesting thing is that the body of the infant is not just the body that belongs to it, but is also the body of its mother taking care of it that is being introjected and somehow being enacted in the mobility of its corporal scheme. To illustrate this point, she gave an example of a child that runs into a desk. The child then caresses its knee using the same gesture that the mother would have used to comfort it. For the child to have replicated this care, already speaks of a certain notion of difference; the infant has introjected an image that splits itself into a body image of a child that is hurt and a body image that caresses it.

That image of the body is structured in the intersubjective relationship between the primary caregiver and the child, so any interruption to that communication would be very traumatic. In the example given before, I spoke of Juarez as a place where femicide is very present, as it is in many other states in Mexico. Only some people in the Republic protest these killings. Some citizens can introject the image of femicide and the image of those women's lives, but to the majority of Mexicans, the image of the women's murders is made abject from the psychic body as if it had nothing to do with them. Even though they are aware of this injustice, there is a deadly instance that makes these femicides unrepresentable to them. The value of otherness is lost when the mechanism of abjection reigns over difference.

Dolto's approach to psychoanalysis in *L'image inconsciente du corps* (1984) is precisely about working with the image of the body, the phantasies that create a particular world of representation. To her, psychoanalysis is about transforming the phantasies that create the image of the body by presenting other realities that have previously been invisible to that body image. After all, as she stated, the image of the body is the bridge with which we communicate with others. To live without an image of the body, we would live in a lonely, silent and narcissistically unstable world. Without words, the image of the body cannot structure symbolism as an archive. It can also be inferred that an appreciation of what is different is necessary to represent bodies (our own and others) and this cannot happen where there is no body image that serves as a bridge for communication The appreciation of what is different includes respecting difference. If difference is understood, the drives of life take up more space for representation, and the death drive does not annihilate the image of the body or the image of others.

For language to make sense in our minds, the corporal scheme must metabolize representations into an image of the body. In Dolto's perspective, one's own name is one of the most important things to metabolize as it secures our narcissistic cohesion. It contributes to the structure of the image of the body. The name is a group of phonemes that accompany human life. It is the signifier of the relationship with the caregiver and plays a central role in our relation to our self and to others. Dolto did not give any examples of this, but I will now introduce an example that I thought of when reading *The Oedipus Plays of Sophocles* (1958). Oedipus in Greek means "swollen foot." When Oedipus was three days old, his parents were told of a prophecy; it said that one day their son would kill his father and marry his mother. In an attempt to thwart the prophecy, his father bound his feet tightly and left him on a mountainside to die. He was found by a shepherd and so survived the ordeal; however, his feet were scarred by this mutilation. The shepherd gave him to King Polybus and Queen Merope who named him Oedipus (swollen foot) and raised him as their own.

Later when Oedipus heard a rumor that he was not the son of Polybus, he went to the Oracle of Delphi to inquire about his birth parents. The Oracle ignored his question, telling him instead of the prophecy that had compelled his parents to abandon him on the mountain. The memory of the representation of his mutilated feet was now attached to the prophecy of parricide and incest. When Oedipus realized that he had fulfilled the prophecy, he gouged his eyes out. Oedipus was the name that held the unity of his body as an archive, but when the somatic energy invested in that body image became a reality, the image of his body as representation broke. This image that condensed the signifiers of swollen feet linked to parricide and incest was contained in his name as a word-representation. The mutilated image of his body brought about the literal mutilation of his eyes attached to the reality of having committed incest and parricide. From this we can conjecture that for psychoanalysis the body image may be a more central concept than the guilt of parricide and incest is in this plot. Oedipus' scarred feet highlight the fact that his body had been marked for suffering since birth. Blinding himself was an enactment of the failure of his name to contain the narcissistic unity of the image of his body. So, in this interpretation of Oedipus, it is not the Freudian Oedipus that is circumscribed in the Oedipal Plot.

Dolto (1984) posits that the image of the body has a narcissistic base image, which is the first component of the image of the body to give the sense of sameness of being. The sense of sameness is a continual feeling of existing, and it keeps a unity between the flesh and a narcissistic image of the body. Sometimes there are failures in narcissism that break this sense of sameness. To her, psychosomatic disorders are an example of authentic failures of narcissism in which death drives localize in regions of the body and cause falls, ulcers, organic attacks, skin disorders. To me, other authentic failures of narcissism happen when people invisibilize themselves and make themselves abject. For Dolto, the narcissistic base image is not only constitutive but is also necessary to relate to other people. Consequently, as others contribute to the base image of the body, failures of narcissism also occur when others make bodies abject. I think it is absolutely necessary that analysts identify when an analysand is replicating the abjection that formed their body and they take care not to collude with this abjection.

Dolto (1984) states that what is constituted in narcissism is the desire to live, therefore to wish that the life of the other is preserved in the projection of our own body image. Narcissism is a symbolic inheritance of the desire of the progenitors that it constitutes a vivid intuition of being in the world. The narcissistic base image cannot be affected or altered without an immediate phantasm emerging. This phantasm is never a pure product of the death drive as the image is already represented. Dolto understands the narcissistic base image as emerging from a representative image of a stage of development. The representative image may be respiratory, olfactory, auditory, or have an oral or anal origin. It returns as a relational architecture that is centered in erogenous places of the somatic surfaces of pleasure. The function of the body image is to link the soma with that which threatens to change the narcissistic base image. We can then say that the body as an archive is constituted by the abjection of what threatens its base image, because, as the representability of this body grows, what has been made abject pushes towards representation. The first comprehension of difference emerges when discerning between one's own image of the body and what the body makes abject, then by understanding that what is made abject belongs to what one does not want to see. To accept and respect difference we have to assimilate what we have made abject as part of ourselves and continue to represent body images even if they threaten our narcissistic base image. To the contrary, the death drive unlinks the representation of our body image and the body image of others so that the acceptance of difference does not occur.

Dolto (1984) also spoke of other kinds of images of the body: functional, erogenous and dynamic. The functional image is an image-movement tending towards the fulfillment of desire. The erogenous image is the one that allows us to feel pleasure and displeasure in response to others. The dynamic image an image in constant movement that exists because the drives of life link the functional image and the erogenous image. Then, the dynamic image corresponds to a fusion of the desire to exist and also desire for the preservation of the life of others. This image allows us to accept changes in ourselves. We can see Dolto's idea as an alternative reading of Freud's conflict between preserving one's own life (self-preservation) and the life of others (conservation of species). The dynamic image allows us to move towards that which we desire. It opens us to the unknown and the unrepresentable. I think that this dynamic image is what enables differences to be respected, as it is through this image, that we prefer to change than to die or to kill. By this, I mean that because of this image the drives of life prevail over the death drive.

This dynamic image is a call to become more than what our body already is. The image of the body is dynamic because in the process of subjectivation when the caregiver disappears, the infant stops crying out for the caregiver. At that moment, the image of the breast morphs into another image of an alternate body or thing that becomes an illusory support. Desire finds a body image that is useful to represent the objects that it strives for; these images change as the image becomes dynamic. Desire strives towards its fulfillment by creating a functional and erogenous image that focalizes its attention on the pleasure it anticipates when obtaining the desired object. The realization of this desire is thwarted when the desire of the subject is insufficient, when the object is absent or when the desire is prohibited.

To Dolto (1984), the erogenous zone can't be introduced to language until it has been deprived of the specific object with which the erotic communication is established. The absence of the caregiver gives meaning to the breast that is lost and also allows for the word-representation of a body image of the mouth. Words become sonorous transitional objects and represent a memory of the image of being an infant linked to the sensation received from the caregiver. This is the child's vessel of communication with its mother and is associated with the phantasm of the first symbiosis.

It is important to my argument to think of the transitional object as a place that is lost and renewed, as we are continually becoming a body. The sonority of the maternal voice at a distance contains the promise of an encounter. The infant experiences a tension while waiting for this promise to be fulfilled; this tension allows it to develop an auditory knowledge of the caregiver's voice. An infant is also a place, the place of the relational bond that is interrupted and recovered. The infant introjects the model by which relational bonds are interrupted and recovered, and these relational bonds continue to re-edit throughout its life. In any stage of development, continuous communication between a body and others allows the images of the body to be renewed so that fragmentation of the body as an archive occurs less frequently. Then, difference is enabled by the dynamic image of the body that allows change in oneself and others.

Dolto spoke of how a symbolic castration delimits tracks of identification with other human beings in order to have a body. Psychoanalysis has used the Oedipal Complex to think of the intricacies involved in symbolic castration. Dolto's way of seeing the Oedipal Complex was that the desiring subject is initiated through a rite of prohibition into the potency of its desire. A law that prohibits incest and parricide is inscribed and offers alternate tracks of identification with other human beings. The adult must not only inscribe the child into the law, but the adult must already be inscribed in it and succumb to it as much as the child. If because of their failures in the Oedipal Complex an adult imposes a law that hurts an infant and enjoys it, we call that adult perverse.

This happens not only between an adult and an infant but in any position where one person is faced with a vulnerable other. Take for example a president using hate speech and eliminating laws that protect people from hate crimes and members of the Mexican government diverting public resources for their personal benefit. This also happens in psychoanalytic practice when we claim that a person's suffering is unanalyzable (unrepresentable) as it does not belong to the Oedipal Plot, and then take pleasure in the image of our own body as normal while considering the unrepresentability of our patients as crazy. This kind of cynicism discourages changes in all bodies as archives; therefore, it is primarily pushed by the death drive. Although not all bodies have had the privilege to be represented and to represent, every body deserves a space with the potential for representability. This is fundamental in the psychoanalytic setting and may seem obvious but is sometimes difficult to put into practice.

It was observation in clinical practice that led Dolto to state that a child who lacks an other that cares for it may get lost inside the mirror as Narcissus did. For her, it is not only about the scopic function of the mother but about a symbolic interaction that posits that infant's body as a body in the world. The body of the child (as an archive) is organized in the dialectic presence-absence of the mother. The image of the body is elaborated as a security web founded by the language of the caregiver. Oral and anal castrations allow a relative individuation, which permits the corporal scheme of the child to break away from that of its caregiver.

As reviewed in Bick's *The Experience of the Skin in Early Object-Relations* (1968) and Anzieu's *The Skin Ego* (1989), the individuation of that pre-egoical narcissism refers to the limits of the skin that emerge from another kind of experience: the experience of the mirror. This occurs when an infant sees or listens to an image (visual or sonorous). Voice and being visible to the other gives the infant the notion that it is the cause of those images. It could be experienced as "I am the presence by which I appear." That presence becomes concomitant of its own presence. The presence of the image is a call as it is directed towards someone. For the body as an archive to become, the body listens to its own voice. In this sense, it is an alienating image if the infant does not have someone around that it can recognize.

Dolto (1984) stated that before the experience of the mirror, the body of the mother or caregiver gives a sense of reference to the primal narcissism of the child. In the experience of the mirror, the image of the body gives form to the infant's own corporal scheme. The infant discovers the joyous character of the image only if its narcissism is satisfied with the image in the mirror. This is the moment of the apparition of the primal identification. Years later, in relation to others and the experience of nakedness, the child's body receives a symbolic assumption to assimilate a sense of embarrassment or need for discretion regarding nudity. The body as an archive assimilates the importance of uncovering itself only under certain circumstances because it recognizes vulnerability and vulnerability appears as dangerous. From then on, the subject is able to see the vulnerability of others. An account of corporal difference allows the child to assimilate with pride (or shame) how it perceives itself. This depends not only on the vision of the body of others but is also referenced to the family's desire for the child, its place in the series of brothers and sisters and the relative importance put on what it is like to be inscribed in a certain place in that family. If the infant does not introject the value it has to its own family; later it will be difficult for the infant to value others.

9

CONCLUSIONS ABOUT BODY FORMATION

In the previous chapter, I detailed what the concept of body is in psychoanalysis and explained that to become a body, we use psychic mechanisms where forms of abjection are produced. I began by revisiting the psychic mechanisms by which a body forms itself as a cultural and political archive. The body is fractured and constantly open to something other than the narcissistic image it holds of itself. It is never complete, and this is what allows the unconscious to speak through us. The body is constantly faced with images from the unconscious in order to keep on representing them.

In Part I, my critical reading of the perspective of different authors offers a renewed metapsychology of the body. To me, it is of primal importance to emphasize how bodily formation is an iterated process that posits human bodies as political archives. We incarnate the problems of our time; therefore, the process of becoming a body is a political process. Not only does power act upon subjectivity, but power and culture contour the very process by which the soma acquires an image of itself to become a body as an archive. Culture is the condition of our agency as bodies, but it also limits that agency. The theory of corporeality given in Part I proposes that although psychic symptoms may appear to be individual, they are primarily political. This argument reveals that the body is an archive of cultural and political practices that does not entirely belong to us yet is constantly acting upon us. In other words, bodies are affected by a set of cultural and political practices, and as a result, there is always an unconscious element to our acts.

The theory I have stated so far is not only relevant in clinical practice but also as speculative theory that sheds light on current political problems. Understanding how a body becomes a body in culture then explains how culture acts as a non-critical dimension of our moral and political deliberations. Thinking of the iterated problem of becoming a body may help us explore the margins of emancipation and political difference. Part I also gives an account of how abjection plays an essential role in the formation of the body. This subject is relevant to the discussion of political problems related to exclusion such as racism, sexism, and classism and must be considered if we are to imagine a different future for alterity.

In Part II I will continue to unravel the difficulty inherent of having a body under the cultural constructions of our time. I discuss how the Oedipal Plot is acting as the hegemonic logic of power par excellence. I give examples of actual social phenomena and present a clinical case that exemplifies that the Oedipus Emplotment makes some bodies abject. A general review of metapsychology and these examples reveal both the iterated problem of being a body in our time and the epochal crisis that is emerging from our interaction with culture.

PART II

Readdressing Oedipus

10

THE OEDIPAL COMPLEX AND THE OEDIPAL MYTH

The Oedipal myth, the complex and its disciplinary normalization

Freud was the master of his own interpretative method; his geniality can be seen in his invention of a method of thinking about bodies that used a tragedy to explain human suffering. He invented a new form of understanding origins where the modern subject was a hero of a tragedy. Freud understood humans to be actors in a multi-generational story while unaware of their role in it. He meticulously sought out examples of the expression of the unconscious in the Western culture of his time. The Oedipal Complex is Freud's reading of the myth of Oedipus as an unconscious element that dominates human life. To Freud, this myth is a tragedy that represents the unconscious life acting over who we imagine ourselves to be; that which exceeds the limits of our consciousness and sometimes acts out.

Freud envisioned the Oedipal Complex to be a universal matrix that explains how psychic life works. In *Three Essays on the Theory of Sexuality* (1905) Freud defined the Oedipal Complex as the organized group of ambivalent desires (love and aggression) that the infant experiences towards its parents during the phallic stage (3–5 years). Although this phallic stage happens during infancy, the complex works silently during the latency period and is re-lived during puberty. It is only then that it is repressed. To Freud, the avatars of this complex are fundamental not only to the orientation of human desire but the structure of the personality as well.

From his interpretation of the tragedy of *Oedipus Rex*, Freud created what I call an Oedipal Plot: a universalizing storyline in which the tragedy works as the unconscious narrative that reflects the human condition and orders kinship and sexual difference. Making Freud's hermeneutic interpretation of *Oedipus Rex* a universal matrix has reduced the myth to a complex, a stage of development and a structure of normalization. Instead of working as an interpretative axis, Oedipus has become the foundation of a conceptual architecture and the mechanism of normalization of bodies for that era and ours as well.

Psychoanalysis was founded as a subversive practice that ideally enables subjects to liberate themselves from imposed forms of relating to others (from hegemonic political practices whose restriction impede a subject from attaining what they desire). A consequence of universalizing Oedipus is that it has engendered ways of interpretation that impose an idealized and disciplinary distribution of subjectivity. Psychoanalysts made this complex the main referential axis in psychopathology, and have tried to determine for each pathological type the modalities of its treatment and resolution. The psychiatric models of today inherited these pathological modalities, and they continue to uphold them. In some psychoanalytic perspectives, Oedipus not only influences the structure of personality but depending on the position that the analysand takes in the Oedipal configuration, it indicates when the analysis should end. According to Roudinesco (2015) Oedipus as a sign has been so universalized that disciplines like Psychoanalytic Anthropology affirm the existence of the complex in diverse cultures even those where conjugal families are not predominant.

I think that the Oedipal Plot is only one of the possible emplotments in the process of bodily formation. But for some reason, Freud tried to ensure that the Oedipal Complex was universal even though there may be other ways of representing ourselves. The consequence of making this plot universal is that today, many psychoanalysts think in terms of understanding a subject only through that Oedipal configuration. Even when analysts think of pre-Oedipal configurations, they are configurations that are constricted by the Oedipal Plot. But that configuration is just another form of giving meaning to what is unconscious. If the limits of interpretation rest in a complex and the way of understanding the subject is through that lens, other possibilities of interpretation, and therefore of representing, are constricted.

The Oedipal Plot has become a technology of power. It has created an impasse that has immobilized the conceptual axis that relates to sexuality and alterity. Psychoanalytic experience shows that the plot as a concept sometimes generates abjection in clinical practice, and this presents a theoretical problem. The psychoanalytic discourse was not intended to generate a technology of the ego but asks us as analysts to place ourselves as the object instead of the subject and then to listen in pro of a deliberate subversion of the impending master discourse of culture. If we are to meet this impasse, Oedipus must be readdressed.

Genealogy of Freud's interest in the Oedipal and its posterior theoretical influence

In *Three Essays on the Theory of Sexuality* (1905) Freud transposed the Oedipal Complex as something unconscious of universal occurrence. To better understand why he placed the Oedipal Plot as a fixed matrix of thought, I will begin by tracing a genealogy of Freud's affinity for this myth. Freud's interest in the myth dates back many years before he began thinking about writing his own version of the tragedy. Existing evidence documents how the theme of Oedipus reappeared throughout his life. It would seem as if the tragedy reverberated, echoing in Freud's body as a manifestation of an epochal body to be reinterpreted, as if Oedipus called him to write in a reflexive movement between his body as an archive of his era and the Oedipal myth as an image of his body.

In *Edipo en la Biblioteca de Freud* (2015) Argentinian psychoanalyst José Treszezamsky did some wonderful research on the bibliographic sources that Freud used in his study of the myth of Oedipus. This analyst discovered that Sophocles' *Oedipus Rex* was not the only version of the myth Freud had read. In fact, the sheer number of versions of Oedipus in Freud's possession speaks of his vast interest in this myth. Treszezamsky's research showed that Freud's first encounter with Oedipus was during his school years. In the program of German schools at that time, it was mandatory to study an introductory book on Classic myths and legends: *Most Beautiful Legends of Classical Antiquity* (1838) by Gustav Benjamin Schwab. Schwab dedicated a whole section of the book to the Theban legend. Two of the titles within this book are "Parricide: Oedipus in Thebes" and "Marriage to his Mother." The emphasis given to parricide and incest in this version may have influenced his later writings.

Schwab's telling of this myth begins with the origins of the story of Oedipus. King Laius abducted and raped Chrysippus the beautiful son of Pelops, so Pelops cursed the king. Zeus learned of his crime, and the Oracle of Delphos foretold that a son would be born to Laius and that his son would kill him and take his wife as his own. Laius' transgression introduced a curse that would have long-term consequences for his family, the Labdacus. The myth of Laius introduced the prohibition of pederasty to Greek culture as in punishment for what Laius did to Chrysippus he was doomed to perish by the hand of his own son. However, Oedipus would also have to pay for his father's crime; his punishment was inheriting guilt for his acts and transmitting the broken family ties to his descendants. From that point onwards, the Labdacus and their descendants were condemned not to recognize each other as kin. They would all appear under the signs of abjection, madness, murder and the stain of guilt until the extinction of their *genos*.

This version of the Oedipal myth with its emphasis on incest and parricide is what Freud had on hand as a child, and it may well have inspired his creation of the theory of seduction and human desire. Schwab's version tells that it was the excessive passion of Laius that led to his rape of Chrysippus. This is said to be the result of Laius' difficulty to be inscribed under the laws of Zeus. As Laius acted outside of these laws, there was no psychic contention for his desire and transgression occurred literally. Oedipus inherits the consequences of this traumatic experience and is also punished because his father had broken the laws of Zeus.

I will now interpret this event according to Freud's theory of seduction, which states that the sexual is transmitted from the beginning of life and because it is difficult to bear, it is repressed. In this scene, Laius breaks the laws of Zeus. His transgression speaks of his difficulty to be inscribed in a symbolic order; in other words, his body is abject. Both the trauma of the sexual transgression and abjection of his father's body are transmitted to Oedipus transgenerationally. To me, this is why Oedipus unknowingly transgresses the prohibition of incest and parricide: he repeats what his conscious mind has repressed. Freud's ideas on infantile sexuality caused a great deal of scandal in his era, which is somewhat contradictory given that many children of that time were being exposed in their textbooks to stories that openly spoke of sexual abuse such as Laius' transgression.

It is important to emphasize that Freud did not go searching for Oedipus but that Oedipus was required reading for him in school, and not only Sophocles' Oedipus but also a more modern version of the myth. The question arises of why at that particular time reading this myth was obligatory in German schools in Vienna. French historian Élisabeth Roudinesco in *Freud: In His Time and Ours* (2016) reported that at the end of the 19th century, archaeological excavations localized the ruins of Troy and Mycenae. As a result, Greek tragedies, myths and the concept of excess described in them were very present in Freud's era. The Greek sagas that were being unearthed spoke of the opposition between the laws of gods and the laws of men. She explained that the epochal configuration of those sagas echoed with the great thinkers of that moment and that is why they chose Greek myths to represent the agonies of their time.

Freud's use of Oedipus in his theories showed great insight into what was happening in the modern era, as well as revealing him to be a subject of that time. Roudinesco (2006) described the end of the 19th century as a strange modernity in which a certain patriarchy had fallen. The men of that era were experiencing guilt, albeit unconsciously because they held themselves responsible for that fall. She took the words of Hugo von Hofmannsthal to state that Freud's generation thought of the world as "the monstrous residence of a king that was dead and a god that had not been born." Roudinesco stated that although modern thinkers of his time wanted to dethrone the patriarchal system (the European empire), they were still subject to that system. This ambivalence bore a resemblance to the Oedipal myth. The modern subject was divided like Oedipus between a conscious desire for social change and the unconscious weight of guilt for having committed parricide when patriarchy was displaced.

Although Freud did not invent the patriarchal system of his era, unconsciously he was both a receptacle for and a reproducer of that system. Freud was receptive to the agonies of his time, and in Oedipus he found a myth that reflected the epochal ambivalence towards the patriarchal system, yet that same receptivity caused him to reproduce that patriarchy in his theories. That is, the epochal ambivalence of his era was metaphorized in a myth that became the basis for his understanding of human subjectivity. While Freud sensed how patriarchal structures were in need of change, the patriarchy of his epoch was perpetuated in his universal family romance, the Oedipal Plot.

Freud was first captivated by the story of the Labdacus family in his early youth, and he was soon immersed in his fascination for Oedipus. When he was 17 years old, Freud (1873) mentioned *Oedipus Rex* in *Letter from Sigmund Freud to Emil Fluss,*

March 17. In the letter, he suggested that Fluss read the Greek and Latin classics, especially *Oedipus Rex* by Sophocles. Freud mentioned Oedipus to him again three months later in his famous letter dated June 16, 1873: *On High School*. He told his friend that as part of a school exam he had to do a translation from German to Latin. Freud was given 33 verses of *Oedipus Rex*. His translation received the grade "good," and in his letter to Fluss, he stressed how he had been given the best grade on that subject. Curiously in that same letter, he told his friend to keep his correspondence in case he was to become famous. Freud seemed to intuit that what he had to say on this subject would be transcendent and from that period onward, his will to fame was attached to representing Oedipus.

Reading Freud's texts, we can imagine him as an adolescent writing to his friend Fluss. His letters speak of his desire to succeed, and his yearning for the purest, broadest goals, stronger rivals, and more serious motivations. Freud wrote that he aspired to leave something important to the world. It was this will for transcendence that inspired him to think of bodies as tragic characters instead of bodies as pure biological units. Later, the young man transformed his reading of Oedipus into a concept that became the center of a conceptual architecture used to catalog bodies. Young Freud's will to fame associated with the sign Oedipus would have a profound effect on his theories.

José Treszezamsky (2015) explained how elements in Freud's library show other sources that enriched his understanding of the Oedipal myth. Freud's library contained underlined references in a number of different versions and interpretations of Oedipus, but it was the tragedy of *Oedipus Rex* that especially captured his interest. Freud read *Oedipus Rex* in its original language; he had a copy of it where the only underlined phrase was when Jocasta said:

> Many a man before you in his dreams has shared his mother's bed, but only those who take such things for shadows feel light the weight of life.

Years later, while Freud was studying medicine, he traveled to Paris to train with Charcot. During his stay, he often went to the theater to see the interpretation of *Oedipus Rex* even though the tickets were more expensive than what he could easily afford at that moment of his life. Freud not only saw the play repeatedly in France but also in Germany in the Busch Circus represented by the Deutsche Theater of Berlin. Freud's keen interest in the Oedipus of *Oedipus Rex* was crucial to the formulation of his complete works and may explain his placement of parricide and incest as the only mechanisms that form the body.

According to Treszesamsky (2015) another reference that was used a lot by Freud was *History of Greek Culture* by Carl Jacob Christoph Burckhardt. Treszezamsky mentions that in a section of the book where the author spoke of Chronos castrating Uranus, Freud underlined twice where it said: "the facts that cause special angst in humanity are destiny and death." For Freud, Oedipus was a myth that represented the conflict between a father and a son, and that conflict includes a symbolic castration, which introduces angst in humanity and a deadly human destiny. This idea was also present in the myth of the primal horde in *Totem and Taboo* (1913), *Moses and Monotheism* (1938) and *Dostoevsky and Parricide* (1928). Freud's understanding of power and destiny revolved around the idea of a tyrannical father and a rebellious child who is obliged to kill him. To him, Oedipus was a tragedy of destiny, and it was only later that he circumscribed it specifically to the consequences of incest and parricide.

In *Letter 52* (1896) Freud's interest in human destiny was already present in his theory that preceded the Oedipal Complex when he started to trace his theory of the unconscious. It was during his stay in Paris that his curiosity about a body beyond the biological body emerged. In his first writings, he was interested in how a split between consciousness and unconsciousness exists in bodies. It may be that while watching the play *Oedipus Rex* Freud observed how Oedipus' guilt was the result of an unconscious force and this influenced the formation of his theories on hysteria. Freud somehow intuited that the cultural manifestation of his time was related to the bodily symptoms of hysterical subjects. However, at this time he was studying medicine and not literature. According to Roudinesco (2016), Freud was interested not only in the interpretation of dreams but also in divinatory traditions and tarot cards. Freud's perspective was divided between that of a medical doctor, a vision that observed and restricted bodies to certain nosology, and that of a receptacle of signifiers of an epoch that lived within him. While conserving his role as a physician, Freud also listened to the narratives of his patients and became a spokesman of the world they faced.

In *Letter 71* (1897) Freud drew a parallel between his version of Oedipus and Hamlet. In a letter to his friend Fliess, he explained that he found an Oedipus in the heart of Hamlet. He said Hamlet's scrupulousness was an effect of unconscious guilt. Years later, Freud wrote *Dostoevsky and Parricide*, and he stated that to him, the three greatest masterpieces of literature of all time were *Oedipus the King, Hamlet*, and *The Brothers Karamazov* and they all included parricide and sexual rivalry for a woman. The scene of a son killing his father repeatedly appeared in Freud's works and became the central concept of psychoanalysis.

To Freud, the prohibition of incest and parricide are what form and delineate the body. The *Primal Scene* was conceived from a plot in which Oedipus kills his father and commits incest with his mother. In *Draft L* (1897) and in *From the History of an Infantile Neurosis* (1918) he explained the Primal scene as the vision of a subject, and two others where the subject is excluded from the relation and incestuous and murderous desires stem from that exclusion. In that scenario, the child interprets the world and his body under the sign of Oedipus. In psychoanalysis, the mechanisms by which the child deals with the primal scene create only three types of bodies: *Verdrängung* in neurosis, *Verwerfung* in psychosis, *Verleunung* in perversion. Therefore, as we listen for the mechanisms inherent to one of these three structures, psychoanalysts turn a deaf ear to whatever else may emerge that is not Oedipal. This is why the Oedipal Plot, may impede our listening to new forms of being a body or bodies in transition from one epochal matrix to another.

The concept of prohibition in psychoanalysis is explained through the prohibition of only two representations: incest and parricide. But as we know, something else always escapes representation, and that is the unconscious. What are the unconscious prohibitions that do not manifest when the prohibition is named either incest or parricide? I state that it is not that these two prohibitions are unimportant, but that they may or may not be central depending on the epochal construction of the body. This is because Oedipus is already a representation but not necessarily the main representation that enables the genesis of drives.

Freud's theory contains a hermeneutical problem: as a man of his time he was called by the themes of incest and parricide and he conferred on them a timeless universality. Conferring universality to the Oedipal Complex meant the only prohibitions that regulated bodies would be a product of both prohibitions. If we consider that incestuous and murderous desires are what is repressed, those themes are already very difficult to think of. What is surprising is that it seems as though to Freud it was less difficult to think in those terms than in other concepts in his works that appear to have been influenced by the myth such as drives, erogenous masochism, bodily formation and primary mechanisms of bodily formation. Revising these concepts may dismantle the problem of universality within the Oedipal Plot. I think that returning to Freud's first theoretical approach to the body before he introduced the Oedipal Plot, may lead us in the direction of new possibilities. A thorough revision of Freud's theory of bodily formation by way of representations and drives may reveal a way to avoid the constrictions that enable difference, as what we have made abject is unconscious and perhaps not even Oedipal.

Oedipus: a mythical representation of an unconscious plot

To Roudinesco (2016), the return to the gods and heroes of Ancient Greece of German Romanticism influenced the Freudian theory of dreams and mobilized questions about the unconscious. The idea of something coming along that overturns everything we think we know was very present for Freud. In *Letter dated November 27 1893 from Extracts from the Fliess Papers*, Freud (1893) quoted an anonymous author: "with frequency, he who looks for something discovers more than what he would want to." Five years later, in *Letter dated August 31, 1899 from Extracts from the Fliess Papers* (1899) he wrote again to Fliess saying that a seeker often finds more than what he wishes for. This idea was of fundamental importance to the Oedipal tragedy as Oedipus led an investigation of the murder of Laius unaware of the role he had played in his father's death.

The same idea is seen in *On Narcissism* (1914) when Freud spoke of the narcissistic object choice: "… psychoanalytic research has revealed a second type, which we were not prepared for finding." This statement of Freud's is concordant with the unconscious being something that escapes spontaneous and reflexive consciousness. His theory of the unconscious was also based on observations of failures of speech; omissions, slips, stumbles or silences that break the logic of continuity of thought and everyday behavior in a way that is incomprehensible. He discovered the significance of these failures while studying the manifestations in hysterical bodies.

For traditional psychiatry, anything that was not conscious was a somatic function; for example, the heart beating or the nails growing. But the Freudian hypothesis of the unconscious introduced a concept of the body that was not only a somatic unity but a body as an archive, that is, a body beyond biology. The discovery of the unconscious indicated a split in the subject. This split is the foundation of the body, a body whose psychic reality is attached to its material corporeality. According to Roudinesco (2016) the ripple of Freud's theory of the unconscious related to Oedipus assured him a place in the history of Western thought. Today it is common usage to say that we did something unconsciously when we do something that is incomprehensible. Freud's writings on the subject of the unconscious created a whole matrix of thought. This Freudian matrix had an impact on how bodies are thought of as being limited by historical representations that are not always conscious. These bodies are an archive emerging from dreams, as the existence of dreams and the unconscious reveals a body beyond the soma. This is the body that I am referring to throughout this book.

In *Letter from Freud to Fliess, October 15* (1897), when Freud was 41 years old, he wrote the first draft of what he would later call the Oedipal Complex:

> Being totally honest with oneself is a good exercise. A single idea of general value dawned on me. I have found, in my own case too, [the phenomenon of] being in love with my mother and jealous of my father, and I now consider it a universal event in early childhood, even if not so early as in children who have been made hysterical. (Similar to the invention of parentage [family romance] in paranoia—heroes, founders of religion). If this is so, we can understand the gripping power of *Oedipus Rex*, in spite of all the objections that reason raises against the presupposition of fate; and we can understand why the later "drama of fate" was bound to fail so miserably. Our feelings rise against any arbitrary individual compulsion, such as is presupposed in Die Ahnfrau; but the Greek legend seizes upon a compulsion, which everyone recognizes because he senses its existence within himself. Everyone in the audience was once a budding Oedipus in fantasy, and each recoils in horror from the dream fulfillment here transplanted into reality, with the full quantity of repression which separates his infantile state from his present one.

In this letter, Freud is analyzing himself, but this act of auto-analysis contradicts his own theory that says the unconscious is inaccessible to us and can only be observed when someone else listens to what escapes from our consciousness. In his letter, Freud says that by himself he could consciously represent an idea (the Oedipal Complex). This is a strange assertion because if Freud was able to represent the Oedipal Complex consciously, then it is not an unconscious element. Therefore, at the core of the concept of the Oedipal Complex, there is an incongruence regarding the unconscious.

Freud not only delimited the unconscious to an Oedipal Plot in this letter but where he said, "Being totally honest with oneself is a good exercise" he appears to be saying that it is possible to be completely honest with ourselves. Freud's illusion of being totally honest contradicts his theory of the unconscious as he also stated that the unconscious is inapprehensible. This speaks of him having a certain difficulty recognizing the primary split that allows the unconscious to exist. I think that what is self-censored in Freud's quote is that in fact we cannot be completely honest with ourselves. As I have pointed out, the primal alienation that is necessary to become a body is so traumatic that we cannot be completely honest with ourselves as we repress the full impact of the truth. What is interesting to me is that Freud could consciously represent the Oedipal Plot. That he was able to represent it would imply that the Oedipal was a truth he could bear. But the unconscious, by definition, is repressed as it is unbearable. How then could Freud state that that which is unconscious is the Oedipal? By stating that the Oedipal Complex is the unconscious plot par excellence, he was again affirming that one can be completely honest with oneself. That is, he did not accept that there may be other plots that escape our cognoscibility.

Although the Oedipal Plot emerged with certain issues, it also enabled a way of interpreting what had been in unconscious in that era. Freud's work enabled a way of interpreting art, culture and symptoms. This is why to André Green (2011), psychoanalysis is a discipline that does not look for exterior validation of its operative field. Freud searched in artwork and myths for material that was useful for interpretation. Some people think that the period of psychoanalytic investigation based on cultural productions, myths or works of art must come to an end. To them, this is because psychoanalysis should solely be the place of listening to bodies. But I have said that bodies are archives of cultural memory and so are myths and works of art. This is why I think that not only do we need to listen to what today's bodies are announcing, but we must also reconsider Freud's placement of the Oedipal Plot as the only normative emplotment in psychoanalytic theory.

On dismantling the Oedipal sign

When interviewed about her biography of Freud, Élisabeth Roudinesco (2015) said that Freud made us heroes of our own lives. A century ago a body in psychic pain would either suffer in silence or be sent to a sanatorium where they were treated as an insane person. Freud saw a resemblance between their situation and a tragedy and instead of confining these bodies, he worked with the literary metaphor of Oedipus to alleviate their suffering. To Roudinesco (2015) Freud's genius was not in founding the Oedipal psychology that is used today to explain everything and its opposite, but because of his gesture to understand every modern neurotic as a tragic character: Hamlet or Oedipus. This gesture of listening to bodies as archives of a tragedy that has meaning must be restored instead of the contemporary reductionism that transforms every human into a chemical machine: a body devoid of meaning.

In the same interview, Roudinesco mentioned something that I find both fascinating and horrible. She spoke of how we as analysts do not always live up to the task of listening. Today, listening to bodies under the Oedipal sign restricts the act of listening and has made Oedipus a normative ideal. What part of the psychoanalytic community does now with the Oedipal is entirely different from the intention it was created for by Freud. Roudinesco's injunction is profoundly assertive, and it invites us to question even the crucial concepts of psychoanalysis today so that psychoanalysis can recover its spirit of liberation of the subject.

Freud's conception of the Oedipal Complex gave an account of the bodies of his time's response to the downfall of a certain patriarchy. His conception became a motionless position in psychoanalytic thought, a matrix that modulates bodies in another representation of a patriarchal system that makes some bodies abject. The problem is that a body today is not the same as a body in Freud's era. The immobility of Oedipus as a sign impedes psychoanalytic listening and is contributing to the difficulty of today's bodies to transform into something different.

The Oedipal Complex gave a phenomenological approach that explained how bodies are normally configured in a patriarchal system. However, through the return of the unconscious many different body images than those considered to be "normal" are represented. By revising Butler's idea on abjection in *Bodies that Matter* (1993), we can see how societal ideals of what a body should be, legitimize if a body matters or not in the world. Abjection is what enables a subject to maintain the illusion of a body. This mechanism entails expelling those who do not fit in the Oedipal scheme to preserve the illusion of being a body that matters. However, abject bodies are agents of a truth that exceeds the Oedipal Plot. These bodies manifest an unconscious image of the body that returns to question culture's ideals.

Oedipus as a sign has generated a discourse that attempts to legitimize what psychoanalysts listen to and what is not to be listened to. It is a coercive form that normalizes what constitutes a valid body and even who is worthy of being analyzed. The idea that a certain ideal of what a body is supposed to be determines analyzability is absurd. If new representations of a body are constituted through the return of unconscious images of the body, then anyone should be analyzable, and the task of the analyst is to listen to any and all unconscious images.

Psychoanalytic practice has showed us that the work of listening is a challenging task, as we never know what may emerge from the unconscious. Assuming that whatever emerges is always Oedipal allows a sense of security, but does nothing to enable difference. In fact, it promotes abjection of whatever appears that is different from the Oedipal Plot, which is very different from the spirit with which psychoanalysis began. Images of the body may change over time through performativity of language, and if these images are changing we have to avoid making them abject; otherwise, the notion of alterity of the analyst will be erased. Freud did something wonderful in his time, which was to listen to bodies. Only if the analysand is a separate other can they be listened to; if the analyst is incapable of perceiving otherness, they will not be up to the task of listening. Today, this act of listening must still be more central to psychoanalysis than any particular plot, so that it enables the subject to represent a space beyond a technology of the ego. If listening is made paramount, then analysis is an act of liberation, a space for fluidity that is committed to listening for the changes in representation of different epochs.

Let us remember that it is the unconscious that resists the master discourse. It was the return of the unconscious manifest in hysterical bodies of his time that made Freud think of new forms of practicing care of the self. The unconscious returns, manifesting itself especially in those bodies that have been made abject. Those bodies are made abject precisely because they are acting out what our unconscious images of the body are. The Oedipal Plot has created immobile ideals of masculinity and femininity and fixed categories that correspond to bodies in pain: psychosis, neurosis and perversion. Abject bodies resist the constrictions of such immobility. Different cultures have had other images of the body to understand sexual difference that are not binary, and patriarchy has made those images abject. Diverse ways of representing difference return from the unconscious to become legitimate again. The Oedipal must be displaced from its privilege as a representation in that conceptual architecture, as it has become an obstruction to listening and limits bodies to certain ideals. On the one hand psychoanalytic theory privileges the discourse of the analysand, but on the other hand it has privileged the Oedipal Plot as the only way of listening to the structural psychic mechanisms.

The task of listening in psychoanalysis is made more difficult because the Oedipal Plot appears as a deaf repetition that disallows the inclusion of new bodily formations. In that same interview, Roudinesco (2015) states:

> When a psychoanalyst tells me that homoparental families are a contradiction to the Oedipal complex, I answer them: Well, then let's change the Oedipal complex for another myth.

We certainly could create other myths to destabilize Oedipus as a sign, but this revolutionary aspiration would then also be responsible for the return of the sign after its erasure. Oedipus has already configured the ideals that determine which bodies are considered normal and which are thought of as abject. The way the Oedipal Plot reiterates abjection is a problem within psychoanalytic theory. The consequences of making Oedipus the architectural foundation of the edifice of psychoanalysis must now be dealt with. However, making Oedipus abject from theory would only create more abjection. Because the Oedipal Plot has formed today's bodies, eliminating it would cause Oedipus to return ferociously from the unconscious. Not only has the Oedipal Plot made some bodies abject, but also some of the components of the original myth. One way to expand the possibilities for bodily formation without inviting the retaliation of Oedipus would be by incorporating other elements of the myth in psychoanalysis.

British psychoanalyst Wilfred Bion said in *Attention and Intepretation* (1970) that analyst's listening should be without memory or desire. But as I stated earlier, as bodies we are archives of memory, and we have been inscribed in or made abject by a patriarchal system where the Oedipal Plot has predominated. Then, to represent other possibilities beyond this plot, more work needs to be done to rethink it and therefore to listen. Freud's theorizations on corporeality allow us to think of bodies as primarily vulnerable to others and an analyst as that figure who takes on the task of listening to that vulnerability. But in the middle of this listening, Oedipus and its consequences are functioning as a master discourse through which we are listening.

If Oedipus is thought of only within the limits of repetition of the plot without difference, the act of listening disappears and bodies become mechanically inserted in a constricting discourse. Listening needs to be inserted into an ethical relationship where the analyst privileges what the patient has to say and questions the crucial concepts that restrict us from listening without memory and desire. Then, psychoanalysis in practice is a work of displacement of prejudice while in front of a body that suffers, a body that has been relegated from speech. To me, psychoanalysis is also the act of attaching that body to its place within language and within its codes of becoming, and this requires going beyond the Oedipal Plot.

In *A Note upon the "Mystic Writing-Pad"* Freud (1925) explained how any mnemic trace is recorded as unconscious memory in any subject; therefore we can say that cultural memory is inevitably affecting the analyst as well. How then can an analyst go beyond the cultural pact of immobility that locks the image of the body into a certain form of patriarchy that has been represented by the Oedipal Plot? Although psychoanalysis emerged as a rebellion against constricting bodies to a medical discourse and as a form of liberation through speech it inadvertently perpetuated certain forms of power.

Psychoanalytic practice is a way of listening to words and images behind what is consciously intended by the patient. The act of listening and interpreting allows new images of the body to emerge. Then it is pertinent to defend psychoanalysis today, as it is a form of care of the self. Freud, when faced with an epochal crisis of the body, did the work of thinking of bodies beyond the concepts of his time. The Oedipal Plot worked in his time, but it doesn't always now. Today psychoanalysis is no longer a predominant technology of the ego. This may be so precisely because the conceptual architecture of psychoanalysis took the sign of Oedipus as its foundation. That which is not identifiable in abject bodies and so resists the sign of Oedipus, announces the existence of a subject that until now has been beyond the analyst's capacity to listen. I think that we should think of bodies beyond the Oedipal Plot as Freud did when he thought of bodies beyond the notions of his time.

Not only did Freud place Oedipus as a central conflict, but he also stated that obedience to the concept (as law) was a statute that legitimizes who may call themselves psychoanalysts. In *Three Essays on the Theory of Sexuality* (1905) he wrote:

> With the progress of psychoanalytic studies the importance of the Oedipus complex has become more and more clearly evident; its recognition has become the shibboleth that distinguishes the adherents of psychoanalysis from its opponents.

Freud's placement of the Oedipus complex as the shibboleth that distinguishes friends from foes of psychoanalysis puts this work outside the limits of psychoanalytic ideals. However, if our loyalty lies in listening to the suffering of our patients, it is necessary to reconsider the immobility of this concept. We may even use Freudian theory to refute the centrality of the Oedipal Plot. If we can ask how a body constitutes itself when facing what it makes abject, we can also ask how psychoanalysis constitutes itself when facing the bodies that do not conform to the Oedipal ideals.

Now is a good time to demystify the myth of Oedipus that psychoanalysis constructed; that is, for the Oedipal Plot of our contemporaries to be demystified, not the Oedipus of Sophocles. A dumbing down has occurred of the concept, caused by the diffusion of a psychoanalysis that has been influenced by culturalism and psychology, that reduces Oedipus to a cartoon of a family configuration. As Argentinian psychoanalyst Nestor Braunstein (2016) said, "let us take out the rind of a simplifying psychoanalysis." The Oedipal Complex has become a sort of manifest content or a phantasmagoria: that which must be crossed out or cleared up.

Freud's Oedipal Plot, in a sense, is the originary trauma of the configuration of today's bodies. The equivalence between the term "Oedipal Complex" and its use at the end of Freud's theory as "Nuclear Complex," already speaks of that trauma. Freud's Oedipal Plot repeated the trauma of a patriarchal system imposing itself over bodies. Today other bodily formations appear that are different from those in Freud's era. They represent unconscious plots beyond the Oedipal Plot and are announcing new ideals. I hope that what emerges to represent these new bodies stays fluid and does not become a position that disables movement of the dynamic image of the body. Freud's Oedipal Plot has been a useful tool for interpretation, but sometimes it may also be a glass ceiling that restricts further modalities of becoming a body. If we are going to readdress Oedipus, different aspects of the sign need to be considered: the deadly reiteration of the myth in psychoanalytic theory, and what bodies that have been excluded from the Oedipal are manifesting.

The often-heard pronouncement that today's pathologies are narcissistic because those bodies do not correspond entirely to the Oedipal Complex posits the Oedipal Complex as privileged as well. This "privilege" given to the Oedipal favors certain individuals at the expense of others and means that psychoanalytic listening actively disadvantages specific groups. Bodies need ideals. Patriarchy had attached a certain ideal of what bodies are supposed to be. Those ideals are presently in a downfall. It is important that these ideals change so new bodies can emerge, but the process of representing our bodies and making new ideals is difficult. If we consider the narcissism of contemporary bodies to be pathological, we may pander to an absurd psychology that writes off whole generations with opinions such as: "Millennials are a generation of narcissists because they take so many selfies." Listening as Freud did for what is being expressed by the epochal body, instead of interpreting it as pathology, might reveal that the process required for the dynamic image of the body to work towards difference involves the body being self-centered. Could it be that while the epochal body is searching for new ideals, it focuses in on itself as it looks to represent images of the body beyond those of the Oedipal sign?

I have mentioned that Freud's psychoanalytic method involved listening carefully to the bodies of his time. His dedication to listening was what allowed him to identify an unconscious plot that represented those bodies in a common cultural background. It has clearly been easier for those of us who work as psychoanalysts to proceed with obedience to the Oedipal Plot and not to have to find unconscious plots relevant to the common cultural background of today. Psychoanalysis needs to overcome abjection and struggle for difference to continue the process of thinking bodies. Bodies today may be formed by new ideals that are different from the Oedipal Plot. Constricting bodies to ideals that are falling can be damaging to them. The deathly repetition of the Oedipus sign points towards either the destruction of psychoanalysis or of the subjects it denies in a practice of exclusion of what it considers normal in the face of the Oedipal Plot.

Has the placement of the sign of Oedipus as immovable law caused psychoanalysis to lose its complexity and is the practice at risk of disappearing because of this? If a coercive force within psychoanalysis makes some bodies abject, the practice is diminished. Instead of rising to the challenge of listening, psychoanalysis merely attempts to master the subject. If we are to preserve the spirit of liberation of the subject that psychoanalysis was founded on, I assert that the best use of Oedipus and its reiteration in psychoanalytic theory is not to remove Oedipus as a sign but to work with the restrictions of the reiterative force that concept of Oedipus has inflicted. To do this we would have to not only think within and outside of the Oedipal Plot, but to think of Oedipus beyond what Freud wrote about the myth, including the many Oedipal themes beyond incest and parricide.

Freeing Oedipus from repetition compulsion

Oedipus as a theme beyond what has been noted in psychoanalysis is a wider and more fertile field of study than incest and parricide. Other themes could enrich the use of this myth in the psychoanalytic field. According to Preciado in *Inappropriate Bodies* (2014) new myths about the body must be created and that the epistemic crisis of the body today should be considered using a genealogy of power. Before proceeding to look for other myths that relate to bodies, let's turn directly to Oedipus and rethink the concept that has been reiterated with very few differences in psychoanalytic theory. Finding different ways to interpret the myth and terminating the reiterations of Freud's interpretation, may free Oedipus from the vice of repetition compulsion that made it an immobile ideal. Reinventing the Oedipal Plot is supplementary to creating new myths and may allow us to expand the field of representability of bodies and sexual difference. To this end, I propose that we focus on Oedipus towards his place of death.

In Sophocles' *Oedipus at Colonus* (1958 edition) Oedipus no longer questions why he killed his father or committed incest, the essential dilemma for him becomes where he will be buried after he dies. That Oedipus cannot find a resting place for his dismembered body is the projection of an image of his broken body. Oedipus' dilemma comes after he faces the main Freudian themes that influence the formation of morality: incest and murder. In his Oedipal Plot, Freud placed these transgressions as central to the foundations of culture and morals. Wouldn't the question of having a place (body) be more central?

Antigone, daughter, and sister of Oedipus, inherits guilt as a consequence of being part of Oedipus' kinship. She commits suicide soon after being placed in a cave to die. The death of Antigone may be a transgenerational re-edition of the difficulty to have a body, and as with some bodies today, the image of the body found no way to be represented. Having a body is a continual process of becoming towards the place of death. The body struggles towards difference, and the only inevitable condition of the corporeal constitution of the human is that it will die. I will do a revision of *Oedipus at Colonus* as it allows us to see how the death drive is at the core of the reiterated problem of becoming a body.

I will now speak of the concept of difference used by Freud in his Oedipal Plot and offer an alternative for the meaning of this concept. Later on I will return to the subject of *Oedipus at Colonus* and its relation to the death drive and bodily formation.

11

RETHINKING SEXUAL DIFFERENCE AND THE OEDIPAL COMPLEX

Sexual difference refers to recognition by the child of the difference between the sexes. To psychoanalysis, this recognition is related to the Oedipal Complex. In Freudian theory, when children acknowledge sexual difference they unconsciously identify with a way of becoming a body (as an archive) in dualistic terms: either masculine or feminine. The difference of sexes as Freud thought of it in *Some Psychical Consequences of the Anatomical Distinction between the Sexes* (1925) is enabled by an anatomic difference between men and women represented by the penis where men have it, and women do not.

At the same time, the meanings and significance which we attach to our materiality do not float free of that materiality of the body. As defined before by Preciado in *Somatheque* (2012) and in *Inappropriate Bodies* (2014), the body is a somatic-psychic archive that contains political, historical and cultural practices. To psychoanalysis, it is only by being bodies that we represent sexual difference and identify with others or not. Thinking along these lines, we could even go further to say that the categories of men and women are a historical construct that has enabled only two forms of becoming a sexed body in the domain of intelligibility.

Even if Freud was trying to understand women by theorizing a general psychology of female sexuality, women appeared as very abstract bodies in Freud's texts. Women were (and still are) associated with what appears as unthinkable or untamable, as those who according to Freud in *Some Psychical Consequences of the Anatomical Distinction between the Sexes* (1927), have an inexorable and impersonal super-ego. The category of women exists and therefore is intelligible, but categorizing women as an ontological failure has rendered them unintelligible to patriarchy. No wonder more women presented hysterical symptoms than men! What is unintelligible to patriarchy or what is unconscious returns from the repressed to speak distortedly through symptoms.

From early days of Freud's writing, he complained about the obscurity enveloping the sexual life of women. The Oedipal Complex gave a clear description of what happens in male sexuality but not in the case of female sexuality. Freud's portrayal of the end of the male child's Oedipal Complex in *The Dissolution of the Oedipus Complex* (1924) gives an account of how men repress their incestuous and murderous desires. This repression is constitutive of the body as an archive. In this way, males become bodies under the domain of intelligibility, but in the case of female bodies, the end of the Oedipal Complex is not as clear.

Addressing the problem of unintelligibility of some bodies in psychoanalytic theory has required an in-depth study of sexual difference and the Oedipal Complex. I will speak about Freud's theory of the Oedipal Complex, sexual difference, representability of men and women, and about the unconscious as the domain of unintelligibility from where other forms of becoming a sexed body that are not heteronormative may emerge. I will also question what kind of sexual difference psychoanalysis is referring to if such differences make other impending forms of becoming a body abject.

In Freudian theory, noticing sexual difference happens in the scenario where children see the body of a person that does not correspond to the same sex as their body. Freud stated in *On the Sexual Theories of Children* (1908) that in the beginning children attribute a penis to all people. To Freud, the first image of our bodies before understanding sexual difference is the representation of a body that has a penis. To him, children's understanding of the absence of a penis can only be understood as a castration. That is, sexual difference is enabled by the idea of a violent disappearance of a part of the body. Fear of castration is another theme of Freud's theory of bodily formation and although it had been mentioned and suggested during his first writings it was for the first time defined in *Analysis of a Phobia in a Five-Year-Old Boy* (1909). As the possibility of a body part being ripped away, cut off or stolen, fear of castration implies that the infant has already assimilated having a body. Fear of castration is a re-edition of the loss of the breast now understood as a loss of the penis. In Freud's theory, we can see that the unity of the image of the body of all genders depends on the idea of having a penis. The castration complex implies the primacy of the penis in both sexes, and its narcissistic significance relies on the penis being the leading erogenous zone. According to Freud, a boy's estimate of the value of the penis relies on his inability to imagine a person without a penis to be of equal value to him and therefore the penis is the universal and essential constituent of valor. Freud's idea of difference in *On the Sexual Theories of Children* (1908) connotes a basic precept that all bodies in the domain of representability are essentially male in the beginning. From this basic precept, stems a discourse that states both that there are two sexes and that difference is determined by a male who has a penis and a woman who lacks one.

In *The Interpretation of Dreams* (1900) Freud suggests that the fear of castration is represented symbolically. For example, the threat of castration can be displaced by the fear of becoming blind like Oedipus, by dreaming of becoming bald or by a fear of going to the dentist to have a tooth extracted. The threat of castration may also be enacted, i.e., when a subject has an accident, which transposes the fear of castration into a real threat to the unity of the body. Castration anxiety is a representative of guilt as in Freud's example of fear of madness and of syphilis due to masturbation. To Freud in *Female Sexuality* (1931) this castration complex also has consequences such as penis envy and feelings of inferiority. Unfortunately, none of Freud's hysterical patients could tell him that more than penis envy, what the acute passion of her body expressed was that in spite of the cultural imposition of men's privilege over women, as a woman she mattered in the domain of intelligibility. The women he analyzed did not say literally, "I feel penis envy." This was an interpretation he made since *On Narcissism* (1914) in which he described the development of a masculine ideal in women as "a survival of the boyish nature that they once possessed."

Freud's theory implies that women inherently lack something that men have, and in fact, that was the cultural dictum. So, while his theory is a phenomenological account of what was happening in his time, he stated it as if it were both universal and permanent. So, this particular historical account of gendered bodies derived from the Oedipal Plot puts female bodies in the domain of unintelligibility and lack. However, its very existence as a historical account means this plot is subject to change. Bodies in the domain of unintelligibility resist absolute abjection. Their presence implores that the cruel norms of civilization that dictate what is considered normal be broken down.

Freud proceeded to assign castration anxiety and penis envy as fundamental positions in the development of infantile sexuality, and he outlined the Oedipus complex as universal. In *The Dissolution of the Oedipal Complex* (1924) Freud makes clear that the Oedipal Complex happens in the phallic stage when infantile genital organization takes place. In this organization, the existence of masculinity is reaffirmed, represented symbolically by having a penis, but in the case of women; they are represented by not having this sexual organ. Then it is the absence of a penis that establishes her difference from men. So in Freudian theory, the only signifier of sexual difference is the penis. It states that the common foundation for the development of both girls and boys is the question of having a penis as it works as a representative of that which they had already lost (the breast). Then, having (or not having) a penis is what constitutes them as sexed bodies.

We can also infer from Freud's theory how the castration complex has an impact on narcissism, as anything that threatens the assumption of completeness that having a penis implies is a threat to the image of the body. For the male child, the agent of castration is the father, but the agent of castration in women is not made clear. In *New Introductory Lectures on Psychoanalysis* (1933), to Freud, women are not castrated but feel deprived because they phantasize that their mother did not give them a penis. The castration anxiety establishes the end of the Oedipal conflict in boys but the beginning of it in girls. Apparently, it was easier for Freud to think of the paths that normed male sexuality take than to understand feminine sexuality.

In *Female Sexuality* (1931) Freud suggested that in the female Oedipal Complex, the girl abandons the mother because of a feeling of hate and disappointment at her mother for not giving her a penis. In *The Dissolution of the Oedipal Complex* (1924) he stated that in the male Oedipal Complex, the child renounces taking his mother as a sexual object because of the fear of castration. The boy's castration anxiety initiates the end of the Oedipal crisis. The boy experiences ambivalence between the fear of castration and pleasure until his fear exceeds that pleasure, so the boy renounces his incestuous desires. This repression of incestuous and murderous desires occurs to preserve the unity of his body. The boy identifies with the agent of castration: his father whom he both loves and fears and renounces his desire to eliminate him. The Oedipal conflict ends with this identification, and at that moment, the super-ego is born as an internalized voice of the agent of castration. The super-ego becomes a moral authority within the ego, an internalization of the father figure.

In *Dostoevsky and Parricide* (1928), Freud analyzed his favorite author's murderous desires towards his father. Freud pointed out that the levels of sadism that the super-ego inflict over the ego as a masochistic instance depends on the severity displayed by the father. The male Oedipal Complex works in the same way as the myth of the primal horde in *Totem and Taboo* (1913). Both are understood by Freud to be the starting point of civilization and morality, as they prohibit incest and parricide. They introduce bodies to a certain kinship or family configuration. Freud's explanation of the Darwinian primal horde in *Totem and Taboo* (1913) was that in primitive times the oldest and strongest male dominated the females and as his young approached maturity they were killed or driven out. One day, his offspring united, killed and then ate the father, and took the females for themselves. Eating him became a metaphor for incorporation. When incorporating him, they experienced guilt. When trying to liberate themselves from obedience to his rule, the dimension of guilt emerged with the dictum that prohibited both killing and intercourse with all the women in the clan which brought about exogamy of the young men. These prohibitions are the foundations of religion, ethics, and culture. Freud stated that there would be no religious belief without the feeling of guilt. Therefore to him, the constitution of kinship implies that just by being born, every descendant is already guilty of committing a crime. That is, a newborn confronts us with the idea that we will die before them and therefore in phantasy, they kill us in the same way that we have killed those that came before us.

The Oedipal Plot and the myth of the primal horde in *Totem and Taboo* are two narratives with the same structure in the sense that they speak of how "lesser men" desire incest and parricide and how the repression of such desires constitute culture. What is enigmatic is that Freud tried to make the feminine body intelligible using the same narrative. In *The Interpretation of Dreams* (1900), he gave his first full account of the Oedipal situation. In it, he proposed that there is a parallel between the development of the two sexes. He posed that a girl's first affection is for her father and a boy's first childish desires are towards his mother. But later on, in *The Infantile Genital Organization* (1923), Freud said that we can describe the Oedipal Complex only as it affects the male child and that the corresponding processes in the female are unknown to us. The male Oedipal Complex was very clear to Freud; however, in spite of his continual listening to female patients and theorizing about femininity, women were always to be his dark continent.

As I mentioned in the first chapter on the subject of hysteria, it was the study of the hysterical bodies at *L'Hôpital de la Salpêtrière* in Paris that initiated Freud's thinking about women's bodies. It was not until *Three Essays on the Theory of Sexuality* (1905) that Freud posed a sketch for his general scheme of feminine sexuality. In it, he said that very young girls always have a masculine character and that the excitability of the clitoris must travel to the vagina. This text has been the source of much confusion. For example, Marie Bonaparte convinced Austrian surgeon Josef Halban to transect her clitoris to reposition the clitoral glans closer to the vagina so that she would have an orgasm that would supposedly belong to the feminine domain.

As we can see in *Fragment of an Analysis of a Case of Hysteria* (1905) when Freud took Ida Bauer "Dora" in treatment, she told him that she felt jealousy because her father might be in an intimate relationship with Frau K., who was nursing Dora's father back to health. Freud did not understand why she would feel jealous and asked her how that could be possible as her father did not have sexual relations because he suffered from syphilis. To that question, Dora's response suggested that desire is not about that. According to Serge André (1999) Freud was perplexed by this statement, and he continued to wonder "What does a woman want?"; this was a question he could never answer. Freud concluded that the erotic life of women was veiled by impenetrable obscurity.

Eighteen years later in *The Infantile Genital Organization* (1923), Freud explained that partial drives are unified in women, and a person as a total object is chosen only when sexual organization is established by desiring what he thought was the ultimate goal: reproduction. In other words, he drew an equivalence between genital sexuality and the desire for a baby. We could then say that as he was thinking of female sexuality, the notion of difference appeared intimately linked to reproduction.

A year after he made this assertion, in his text *The Dissolution of the Oedipal Complex* (1924), Freud explained that there are three paths that women may take towards the resolution of this stage. He did not explain the process of repression that ends the Oedipal Complex in women, but in it he described three types of feminine bodies that emerge from these paths. One of these bodies develops a masculinity complex where the girl thinks that the clitoris will grow into a penis. Another manifests a certain kind of asexuality where the girl refuses anything that has to do with genital sexuality. The third body he called femininity, culminates in the girl's desire to give a son to her father. I find it bizarre that Freud only deemed one of three paths that women take to resolve the Oedipal to be feminine. Only in the third option could women attain the category of femininity, by desiring something that men have (the phallus) which in a symbolic equation transposes into having a baby. So, returning to Freud's question "what do women want?" it is as if he surmised "it is something that she lacks and that only men can give her."

Femininity as thought of in Freud's third option would then belong to a sense of property, to the terrain of the Pater Familias. Following Freud's logic, this implies that males renounce their incestuous and murderous desires entirely to leave their family of origin and love a new one, while women do not. Their incestuous connection that desires to give a son to their father makes "feminine" women the caregivers and preservers of kinship and creates connection between the generations. This logic, of course, corresponds to the very intricate problem of patriarchy.

As Preciado stated in *Inappropriate Bodies* (2014), women as a space of reproduction is a modern political fiction that affected their bodies. Before the 18th century, reproduction was thought to take place in the drop of sperm and not within the body; the resulting infant was then a product of men and God. So ontologically speaking, a woman's body was considered a failure. The Word of God that sustained women's uteri fell to immanence as God fell. The uterus would now find no symbolic respite in God and what it meant to be a woman was now open to new possibilities. This posited women as those who would have to take charge of their bodies and rethink the belief that their bodies were an ontological failure. I think that Freud's notion of femininity may have been a proposition that tried to repair this fall of the Pater Familias. On the one hand, by reinstalling a patriarchal model, Freud's notion of femininity restores the figure of the Pater Familias. On the other, stating that femininity as such comprised the women's desire to give a baby to their father suggests that man's exclusive relationship with God lacked the power to engender life.

In *The Formations of the Unconscious* (1958) Jacques Lacan stated a difference between hysterical bodies and feminine bodies and critiqued Freud's attempt to understand women through the lens of masculinity. In his structural approach, the hysterical position is masculine. He defined the feminine position, as the position of love, of giving something that one does not have (symbolically the phallus) to someone who is not (what we represent the other to be). To Lacan, this feminine position of loving meant the subject desires something beyond having a penis. He understood feminine desire to be of an infinite mystical order. In *On Feminine Sexuality: The Limits of Love and Knowledge* (1972) Lacan agreed with Freud's perspective in the sense that sexual difference is recognized only by way of the having or not having the phallus. The phallus is what represents man, and so women are relegated to a place of lacking it. So then, "The Woman" does not exist as women are unrepresentable bodies. To him they use masks to create themselves and incarnate a form that can be taken as the object of desire of others.

Once again, Lacan's perspective points to sexual difference being a sense of property where one has or does not have the phallus. To him, the erogenous sexed body is always crossed by a phantasmatic experience. That is, a body whose materiality has a penis may be a woman if its subjective experience is one of lacking the symbolic phallus. Women may be in a masculine position if their experience is that of having this phallus. But in any case, linking lack to femininity posits sexual difference in terms of representability and unrepresentability. One bodily configuration includes incognoscibility (feminine position), and the other bodily configuration is absolute cognoscibility (phallic or masculine position).

When speaking of sexual difference, Freud and Lacan used the binary categories of masculine and feminine. However, these categories are never free of ideology and history. What is considered masculine and feminine references the symbols and images of gendered figures that prevail in a current cultural domain. If we recognize that a metaphoric function of language enables us to represent our bodies as archives, we need to accept that senses are indistinguishable from the symbolic order that administers the body and therefore perception carries with it a certain ideology. Concepts such as masculinity or femininity could not be empirical or essential entities, but constructions that are associated with becoming a body. However, this does not mean that the categories of masculine and feminine should always remain the same over time. The unconscious will always return and expand the limits of what is cognoscible within the limits of our language.

In both, Freudian and Lacanian theory, the masculine body appears as a body that can represent itself and a feminine body as one that escapes representation, which erases the fact that all bodies are subject to incognoscibility. This definition of sexual difference gives a status of privilege to masculine bodies, favoring an androcratic order. Despite being considered unrepresentable within the order of sexual difference, women are still being named. Naming categories of sexual difference as masculine and feminine establishes a space of representability where other subjectivities or forms of being a body are abject from the cultural domain. Therefore, in psychoanalysis, bodies that are outside the limits of sexual difference that represent this androcratic order are made abject.

As seen in the example of the women of Juarez that I mentioned before, one form of making bodies abject is by not naming them. So, an essential part of accounting for the bodies that the epistemic crisis of today is announcing is naming categories that did not exist before. Examples of such categories are; transgender females, transgender males, intersex nonbinaries, intersex binaries, bi-gendered, androgynous and any other gender identity, gender expression or sexual orientation.

I think that sexual difference must transcend to a differentiation that does not make any human abject. This requires expanding unintelligibility within normed bodies and naming as intelligible those who have been made abject. This could be done in psychoanalysis by changing the Oedipal Plot's phallocentric order. The task of dismantling the psychoanalytic form of understanding sexual difference would be to speak of Oedipus' abjection. This elaboration of his abjection would enable us to name therefore represent a part of what is made abject in ourselves and in society.

When Freud spoke of the phallus as the main organizer of sexual difference in *Three Essays on the Theory of Sexuality* (1905), he also decentralized it when speaking of polymorphous sexuality and the child's ability to find erotic pleasure in any part of its body. The body as an archive represses or disavows unconscious elements, but that does not mean that life is always normed by what is not repressed. Freud could give form to the Oedipal Complex precisely because the forms of being a body it represented were in the domain of intelligibility and not entirely unconscious. Note how the phallus has been taken as the main organizer because it has been a fundamental symbol in the domain of intelligibility.

Because of a certain historical context, Freud thought that the main goal of sexuality was the perpetuation of the species and the creation of a family. According to Preciado in *Inappropriate Bodies* (2014) today, other forms of becoming a sexed body emerge beyond the goal of reproduction. These bodies announce the fall of certain ways of thinking about sexual difference and the body. Technologies such as sex reassignment surgeries and assisted reproduction are in the domain of what is possible today. Such technologies change the limits of cognoscibility and the limits of what is possible for the materiality of bodies. Is it possible that a new order of power may emerge, different from that centered on the phallus? Although right now, the order of power prevalent in the cultural domain is phallocentric, it is necessary to work with that which returns from the unconscious and begin to represent a new order, even if at present, this is a utopia.

The current crisis of the body makes it necessary for psychoanalysis to address how abject bodies can represent themselves if the normative representational path excludes them. Since Freud's time, this normative representational path has been acting upon bodies so that it makes it difficult for abject bodies to represent themselves beyond that normative plot. What further complicates the ability of abject bodies to represent themselves in the cultural domain is the difficulty we all face to appropriate sexuality, as its origin is in the desire of other's implanted in us. Not even men that are represented by the Oedipal Plot can appropriate themselves entirely. As I said in the first part of the book, the body is always struggling to represent itself, and it is precisely in that struggle that the difference between oneself and the world is discovered. Although we live in a shared culture, every body has a very particular experience and relationship with otherness that may correspond to different plots.

In psychoanalysis, representing otherness is what allows difference to appear. Sexual difference needs to be thought of in other ways that do not make those that are not masculine abject. To have a more radical understanding of sexual difference, psychoanalysis should refrain from imposing definitions about what femininity or masculinity means. Sexuality is a particular-plural, it is a re-edition of the sexual and it happens differently in each body.

12

THE BROKEN HOUSE OF LABDACUS, THE BODIES OF STRANGERS AND THE PLACE OF DEATH

So far, I have elaborated an account of Freud's Oedipal Complex as a matrix, which gives limits to the body as an archive. I stressed that the body is built through historical and political narratives and emphasized how in Freud's time many bodies were suffering an epistemic crisis of the body because of the fall of the Pater Familias. I also stated that the way of understanding sexual difference has relied on the difference between masculinity and femininity. In psychoanalysis, one position (masculinity) or the other (femininity) relies on a certain duality determined by the presence of a penis or a lack of it.

Bodies constitute through narrative fictions. The child's perception of sexual difference is already an inseparable part of the narrative fiction that forms the body of the child. *Some Psychical Consequences of the Anatomical Distinction between the Sexes* (1925) allows us to see that as a product of his time Freud's perspective is that if a child is born with a penis, he is a man and if not she is a woman. Also, being a man or a woman implies assuming a certain position of subjectivity. This indicates that the current order of sexual difference establishes a gendered opposition between bodies. Bodies reproduce certain practices within the limits of what is possible for men and women within the cultural domain. This does not mean that our culture's heteronormative order of sexual difference is not subject to change. Today, there are possibilities available to bodies that did not exist before. For example, the availability of sex reassignment surgery and assisted reproduction techniques are changing the limitations of this symbolic order.

To Freud, men's bodies are masculine because of the representation of having a penis. This entails that they represent themselves as having bodies that are complete (not lacking), but as a result, they fear being castrated. This fear threatens the unity of the body. As seen in *The Dissolution of the Oedipus Complex* (1924), men repress whatever threatens the conception of their body as complete. This fiction of a complete body works until the mechanism of repression fails and what was unconscious, what had been unintelligible returns. This implies that masculinity serves as an escape from the most different paradigms of unconscious subjectivity.

In Freud's perspective in *Three Essays* (1905) and in *On the Sexual Theories of Children* (1908), because women do not have a penis they represent themselves as bodies that lack something and envy those with a penis. In *Some Psychical Consequences of the Anatomical Distinction between the Sexes* (1925) he proposed that woman have three responses to this penis envy; believing that they will grow a penis, adopting a certain kind of sexual inhibition or realizing a symbolic equation that replaces the penis with a baby. Freud's approach is a phenomenological description of what he observed in the subjects of his time. For him, femininity works as a metaphor for gratitude, for giving life to the one that created them. However, even if we agree with it as a metaphor, let us take a moment to think of how it places women in a different order of kinship from men. Men are rooted in the family they belong to as sons, they completely renounce their incestuous and murderous desires towards their parents to become a man and create a new family. But women are not only rooted in their family of origin, as their incestuous desires are still directed towards their own family.

According to Freud, femininity means to desire to have a baby for the father. We may then conclude that the ultimate object of women's sexuality is the child or her father instead of her partner. This dynamic puts women in a different and strange symbolic place of kinship where it is unclear whether women are daughters or partners to men. The Oedipal Complex then not only describes a stage of development but points to an existing cultural confusion regarding kinship. Men's place in kinship is well delimited, and women's is not. This disorder in kinship not only mirrors Patriarchy but also perpetuates it.

Freud's theory of feminine repression in *Some Psychical Consequences of the Anatomical Distinction between the Sexes* (1925) states that this mechanism does not happen in such a forceful way as it does in men. This posits feminine bodies as those who are closer to what is unconscious and may be why feminine sexuality always remained an enigma to Freud. We can then say that becoming a feminine body implies that unconscious sexuality exceeds the Oedipal Plot. To me, the Oedipal Plot has defined what bodies are considered legitimate in a Patriarchal culture. As it is a derivative of the dynamic unconscious, it manifests symptomatically. The very fact that this plot is representable makes it intelligible. This plot is not within the unconscious, the domain of unintelligibility. If Freud could use the Oedipal Complex as a metaphor for the development of human sexuality, it is because this complex is of the domain of intelligibility and therefore, is not unconscious today. It would seem as if the bodily formation of masculinity works as an egoical escape from the most different paradigms of the sexual, including the dark continent of femininity. Femininity has taken form as a category of unrepresentability, with women's abjection serving to preserve the representability of men. This is paradigm in itself, as the very existence of a category named woman, means they are representable. Then, bodies that are made unrepresentable by the Oedipal Plot announce by their very existence impending plots and narratives and call for their inclusion.

The binomial categories of gender, male and female, are fictions that have been recurrent in time, and to Freud, they are constitutive and enable representation of the body. The Oedipal Complex circumscribes this representation as a phantasmatic primary scene where the body discovers a specific form of sexual difference. It seems that to Freud men become masculine bodies by repressing fear of castration, whereas women are constantly representing their body as femininity is understood in masculine terms, namely, its lack of a univocal representation (a penis). Freud's ideas on feminity through his texts and condensed in *Female Sexuality* (1932) allows us to see that to him the prohibition of parricide and incest works differently in women than in men. Women's envy (which is murderous) would also need to be repressed, but he did not tell us how that happens. Freud considered a woman's relationship with her mother to be inherently difficult; he described it as both intense and ambivalent. He stated that it is only the daughter's hatred towards the mother for not giving her a penis that allows her to separate from her mother. We could see this as saying that in the female Oedipal Complex, the condition for her to repress incest, is that her murderous desires are enacted in the form of hatred for her mother. It is just after this separation with the mother that those incestuous feelings find another object: the father. To Freud, this object (the father) is chosen because he has what she lacks (a penis). We could then say that in Freud's theory, the incestuous and murderous desires of women are not repressed, but have a phantasmatic realization. In a symbolic equation women give a child to their father (metaphorically), and by way of murderous desires expressed as hate, they separate from their mothers.

According to Freud's theory, when this repression of murderous and incestuous desire does not occur, two other mechanisms enable ways of becoming a body. One of these ways as described in *Psycho-Analytic Notes on an Autobiographical Account of a Case of Paranoia* (1911) is by becoming psychotic, through a mechanism of repudiation, which is a primordial expulsion of the fundamental signifier (phallus). The other as described in *An Outline of Psycho-Analysis* (1938) is by way of perversion, through a mechanism of disavowal that consists of rejecting the perception of women's lack of a penis. These two mechanisms happen in the primal scene and construct abject bodies in the sense that they are in the limits of the Oedipal Plot. By the very definition of their mechanisms, these bodies operate outside of the law that dictates that one shall not kill or commit incest. Therefore, the moral of this symbolic parental law is mediated by the vision of the male sexual organ and not the female sexual organ.

If we take into account the historical context of Freud's time, we could certainly understand that to him women were those who lacked something that men had. However, understanding the context of Freud's ideas does not mean that they should necessarily be given permanence. But as I stated before, in Occidental culture, binary categories of gender have been reiterative in time and have constituted specific ways of being a body in the cultural domain. It is our task to recognize that bodies and categories of gender are in the process of changing today and that these body configurations and gender categories morph and affect each other.

According to Roudinesco in *Freud: In His Time and Ours* (2016) Freud listened to the bodies of his day that suffered an epochal crisis that rendered the image of their bodies unstable. In this sense, he was a hero as the Oedipal Complex could give these bodies symbolic content. Psychoanalytic listening that employed the Freudian plot offered hysterical subjects relief from their suffering. Such is the case of Bertha Pappenheim (Anna O.) whose symptoms disappeared. Moreover, in a context where the epistemic crisis of the body pointed to the difficulty of women to appropriate their bodies, she went on to become an outstanding defender, advocate, and pioneer of women's rights!

Today, many still think of bodies in Freud's binary terms, but this leaves any other way of being a body abject. Even though the Oedipal Plot alleviated symptoms in Freud's time, it would be quite irresponsible if we ignore what is emerging in today's bodies. This abjection establishes in the domain of culture a symbolic law that is outlaw. By this, I mean that although the Oedipal Plot establishes a law that prohibits incest and it does not protect all bodies from being killed. For example, many psychoanalysts hold that trans people are psychotic or perverse because they repudiate or disavow the phallic signifier of sexual difference that conservative psychoanalysis dictates. Wouldn't that perspective itself be the murder of other possible forms of subjectivity beyond the Oedipal Plot?

If new sexualities are emerging from unintelligibility, it is our task to think of them instead of making them abject. There is a big difference between making abject what is not a body, and making bodies abject that already exist and therefore, have the potential to be represented. Some abject bodies may not have the coordinates to represent themselves under the androcentric order of the Oedipal Plot, but this cannot be confused with saying that there are no other possible plots. Abject bodies exist, and to live they push towards representability. By their very existence in the world, these bodies manifest a failure in culture's symbolic domain and therefore a failure in the way the Oedipal Complex works.

War, racism, classism, sexism and a culture of hate is the very proof that today's culture has failed to prohibit incest and murder; its distribution of bodies under categories of sexual difference promotes violence by making abject any body that is not cisgender, heterosexual, white and male. To find an effective injunction that prevents culture from manifesting its incestuous and murderous desires, it is necessary to question the description of bodies in the Oedipal Plot. After all, the essential contribution of the Oedipal Complex is the prohibition of incest and parricide, and today we see how failures of this prohibition appear in the form of war, exploitation, and many other forms of violence. How can culture sustain these prohibitions if it is committing them itself? Our culture's blindness of the violence directed towards abject bodies has generated deadly consequences.

Addressing the status of unrepresentability of abject bodies will require that difference and abjection be restated. One way of changing how difference and abjection are thought of would be by representing other forms of Oedipus as a sign. The rest of this chapter will focus on reinterpreting Oedipus as a figure whose primary dilemma is that he is a stranger within his own kinship and as a consequence, his body is an inhospitable place. Focusing on Oedipus' status as a stranger may help us see how the Oedipal Plot has failed both to give a symbolic account of bodies and difference and to prevent the destruction of parricide and incest. To do this, I will explore the question of what is it to be a stranger. This chapter will also examine the relation between Oedipus' kinship and place of death, and the general incompleteness of bodies. It also explores whether the theme of Oedipus' body as an inhospitable place may be even more primary to the constitution of the body than the prohibition of parricide and incest.

With that in mind, I will now speak of certain elements of the *Theban Plays* (ed. 2003) by Sophocles that focus on the figure of Oedipus and his journey towards his place of death. The Theban dynasty of Labdacus was mainly concerned with the structures of kinship. The Labdacus' family, the Labdacids, included Laius who fathered Oedipus and Oedipus' descendants: Polynices, Eteocles, Antigone, and Ismene. Sophocles wrote Antigone before Oedipus Tyrannus and Oedipus in Colonus even though the events of the play occurred after the death of Oedipus. Following Sophocles' order of time, I will first speak of Antigone in this account of Oedipus towards his place of death.

When Oedipus was disgraced, his sons Polynices and Eteocles were too young to rule, so their uncle Creon served as the regent of Thebes and for a time he shielded the city from the curse that fell over Oedipus' descendants. Once they were of age, Polynices and Eteocles argued over the throne, and Polynices was violently ousted from the city by his brother. In exile, Polynices married the daughter of the king of Argos, and with the king's help, Polynices led an army to attack his homeland. Polynices, son of Oedipus, betrayed his own kinship by bringing strangers to fight with the city of Thebes. He who was estranged from his kinship then sent strangers to battle with them, and it was this confrontation that threatened the unity of the body of the city of Thebes. My reference to the unity of the body of a city is because as I depicted before from Freud's *The Ego and the Id* (1923), the world as we understand it is an extension of the body as an archive.

This threat of castration or destruction of the city was a consequence of Polynices' rupture with a certain order of kinship. However, according to Sophocles' *Theban Plays* (2003 edition) the army of Thebes won the battle and at least in one sense preserved the unity of the city. But in another sense, the unity of Thebes failed, as there were many casualties among their troops, including Megareus (son of Creon). In this battle, Antigone's brothers Polynices and Eteocles fought each other to the death. Afterward, their corpses were marked with a sign on the forehead that signified the transgression of fratricide.

The very meaning of the name Creon is ruler, and as their uncle's body image was strongly attached to his name, an idea of being a sovereign ruler was deeply rooted in him. When Thebes was attacked, not only was the unity of his body threatened but the sovereignty implicit in his name as well. His response to this threat was to decree that all Argean dead were to be left unburied after the battle. It was as if denying them a place reaffirmed his status as respectable king and therefore afforded status to the body of Thebes. Only after Theseus fought Creon in an alliance with the democratic city of Athens, could the bodies of the people of Argos could be buried.

In Sophocles' Antigone in *The Theban Plays* (2003), Creon rewarded Eteocles posthumously for defending Thebes by reinstating him as a citizen worthy of burial and therefore his body was restored its place in kinship. The point of departure of this play is the importance having a place of burial has to kinship. As Eteocles' forehead was marked by fratricide, his corpse ran the risk of being treated as though it were that of a stranger; his burial depended entirely on the uncle Creon's recognition. This part of the tragedy points to after losing someone we may avow or disavow them; avowing them entails that we give them a place to be mourned (represented). Whereas Eteocles received a noble funeral, Polynices received the punishment for traitors and his uncle did not give permission for him to be buried. Creon made a distinction of whom he would avow and whom he would not; this distinction determined who was a stranger and who was part of his kinship.

According to Meineck and Woodruff's Introduction in the *Theban Plays* (2003), in Greek culture not receiving burial was a cruel punishment as it meant that the unburied dead would be shamed and unable to rest and that their family would carry shame as well. This unburied corpse would cause miasma, which to the Greeks was ritual pollution. Miasma implied a curse that spread over the lands and would then mistreat the Labdacids. An unburied corpse would also be an affront to Hades. For Antigone this was unbearable; she sided with divine law when she opposed her uncle Creon and tried to bury her brother. One order of kinship was broken when she ascribed to a more divine order of kinship.

Judith Butler, in *Kinship Trouble in The Bacchae* (2017), was referring to this scene of Antigone when she questioned if failures in kinship happen because one set of ordering relations irrupts into another set of them. She said that such is the case with Antigone as she wanted to honor familial bonds and this caused problems in the order determined by the state. Creon and Antigone were defending different ethical values, both demanding the preservation of a set of ordering relations that was essential to them. While Creon enforced the preservation and unity of the body of the city-state, Antigone defended her family's right to bury their dead, to give a hospitable place to her brother's corpse. For the sake of the living, she wanted to preserve the status of the one who had died. Her link to her brother Polynices was more important to her than her ties to the city-state or family ties of marriage, which are given by law and not by birth. Antigone and Creon had different perspectives on kinship, on whose bodies should be represented or considered to be strangers.

According to the *Theban Plays* (2003) Antigone claimed that the dignity of her brother's body and his place of burial had precedence over the laws of the state and she did not care if they were transgressed to bury him. Antigone tried to convince her sister Ismene to help her, but her sister's ties were to the state, so Antigone herself assumed the task of burying her brother. When the guards of Creon discovered what she was planning, she went to Creon and confessed her intention to break his law: "Nor did I think your orders were so strong that you, a mortal man, could overrun the gods' unwritten and unfailing laws." This act of confession and willingness to confront her uncle put her body at risk, so we can see that although she wanted to appear as sovereign, she could not be. Her words exposed Creon's breakability; she showed him his failed illusion of immortality by saying that he was speaking as if he were a god. By this, she was pointing to the general breakability of bodies and saying that only gods are not broken (are immortal). Antigone speaks in the name of gods and in doing so puts her own life at risk. She denounces the king's breakability; however, her actions decry a lack of awareness of the limits of her own mortality. In addition to being broken, hers was an abject body in the sense that her desire to bury her brother did not receive approval from the state.

Antigone wished to bury her brother so that the symbolic distinction between life and death was preserved. Her passion to give him a proper burial, even if it put her life at risk, was because she could not grasp this distinction. This is evident in her lack of concern for her own body and her absence of fear of the deadly consequences of her actions. Led by a phantasy of immortality that she herself reproached in Creon, she acted in a way that put her life in jeopardy. Later, when Antigone was caught in the act of burying Polynices Creon imprisoned Antigone in a sepulcher. Then, in her place of burial, she hanged herself. Being interred alive became the factual representation of her illusion of immortality, and the impact of this scene was such that her next act was to destroy the materiality of her body. Antigone's suicide put an end to her phantasy of immortality while at the same time was a subversion Creon's authority over her body. The tragic nature of her act speaks of the intensity of the death drive when it finds no respite in a representation of the body.

In *Antigone's Claim: Kinship between Life and Death* (2000), Judith Butler discusses Hegel's interpretation of Antigone. For him, Antigone could not find a place for her body because she was not capable of offering or receiving recognition within the ethical order. The only bond of kinship that Antigone recognized was that with her dead brother. Fraternal unity and blood ties established a certain kind of kinship and an internal dynamic of recognition. To Butler, Antigone's act of subversion was unsuccessful because her representative function was itself in crisis. Her body was inhospitable, as there was no image of the body that sustained her in the world. As I said earlier, the act of representing has been thought of as the symbolic feature that allows for the possibility of becoming a body. In this tragedy, the horizon of intelligibility in which Antigone operates is blurry because a disorder in kinship breaks the symbolic order. Therefore, she remains somewhat unthinkable as a body in the world. Something in the order of her body image is broken. The body image that is broken is a consequence of a broken kinship: the broken house of Labdacus.

In *The Essence of Tragedy* in Seminar VII (1956–1960), Lacan referred to Antigone as essentially beautiful because of her enigmatic character. While alive she was in service to death, and this placed her in the limits between life and death. She fought against Creon, but they were not that dissimilar as both sought a position of sovereignty. It was this pretense of sovereignty that led Antigone to speak in the name of the gods on several occasions. But Lacan's description of Antigone as "essentially beautiful" merits suspicion. This fascination with the beauty in her part of the tragedy masks the nightmarish aspects of what is unrepresentable in Antigone's service to death. We can see the radicality of the death drive manifesting when, by revealing to the king her intention to betray his decree, she sabotaged her own plan thereby assuring she would be condemned and buried alive. *Antigone's Claim: Kinship between Life and Death* (2000) by Judith Butler includes a critical reading of Lacan's appraisal of Antigone. She points to how his perspective disregards that she was committing a crime that would not only be a crime against the state, but would take her love for her brother to the extreme of losing her own life.

We can see a parallel between the figure of Antigone and Freud's understanding of women, as both narratives describe bodies that are archives of a broken kinship. As I have exposed through this book, women in Freud's time manifest the fall of the Pater Familias, while the order of kinship in Antigone's body was broken by her father's transgressions of incest and parricide. Also, Freud's theory states that women want to give a son to their father and Antigone, although betrothed to the son of Creon, chose the quest to bury her brother over a life with her partner (future husband). The image of Antigone's body was broken, and in an attempt to replace it, she identified with a body that was going to be buried without dignity. She preferred to die for love of her brother than to create life in ways that were not as incestuous or murderous. Repression of incest and parricide failed because the symbolic order of her body had failed. This failure was derived from Oedipus' acts, his descendant then inheriting the incapacity to become a body under a familial order. Unlike Freud's Oedipal Plot, here, the prohibitions of parricide and incest were not a result of the guilt of Oedipus but of a disorder in kinship.

As stated by Françoise Dolto in *L'image inconsciente du corps* (1984), to have a place in this world it is of primordial importance that our bodies are granted a certain permission, one that allows us to exist and desire. The first place, where the representation of the body image is enabled, is always a symbolic one. We can see in the *Theban Plays* (2003) that Antigone was disavowed of her place in kinship, so she failed to constitute a body image that protected her in the world. She then put herself in circumstances that endangered her body. Her refusal to obey Creon's decree meant she was buried alive, which can be seen as a metaphor of becoming trapped for eternity. Then, to end her predicament, she hanged herself. This scenario of entrapment speaks of her difficulty to host her body, and therefore to find a hospitable place in the world.

The book *Of Hospitality* (2000), by Jacques Derrida and Anne Dufourmantelle, offers a perspective on what it means to be a stranger and what being hospitable to bodies implies. In this book Derrida explained that there are always three figures in a scene of hospitality: a host, a guest and a witness. To Dufourmantelle, the witness may be a space or a place and not necessarily a body. Derrida considers hospitality to be one of the main laws of culture. To him, language is the key that allows bodies to be symbolically inserted into the laws of hospitality. Laws of hospitality exist because there is also another figure that threatens hospitality: the figure of the parasite. He defines a parasite as one who has entered a place without permission; where there is no host or witness.

In my interpretation, the figure of Antigone is a parasite; not only did she lack permission to bury her brother, but being buried alive meant that she also would have no tomb to witness her death. By defending her brother's right to an official burial, Antigone was fighting for his place; a tomb that would bear witness to his death, and allow him to be a proper guest in the house of the dead. Antigone's fight for her brother to be given a legitimate place was not only motivated by love but also because she herself lacked the status of being a guest in the world. This defense of her brother's right to a burial meant she met the same fate as he did. As I said before in this work, the world is a projection of the body as an archive, and we can see how Antigone's body was broken. Because her body lacked the necessary representation to host her, Antigone's tomb was not a proper witness for her body to be hosted in the world of the dead either. Her body was a body that suffered from uncognoscibility; it was the body of a stranger. She and her brother were strangers whose bodies were not hosted by an architectural witness (a tomb), as tombs are homes for the dead. By losing the possibility of an official burial, they lost not only a tomb but also a metaphorical space to be mourned.

In the same book, Derrida explained that *hostis* is the root of the word hospitality and it is an undecidable that contains both the meanings of hostility and hospitality. Therefore, the parasitic hostile enemy is contained within the word that hosts it. In hospitality, there is a necessary linguistic violence; as a prerequisite to entry, the host asks the person certain pointed questions that will give legitimation to their status as a guest. Who are you? Where do you come from? What is your name? Dufourmantelle then commented that to exist, or using a term I used earlier, to not be a stranger, the subject must have a symbolic place that is recognized by others. So, what are the parameters that afford us a symbolic place of recognition in the eyes of others? And given those parameters of recognition, how can one give an account of a body that is considered to be a stranger?

The way I have referred to the body as an archive entangles it in a dynamic where the body is always at risk of becoming a stranger as it is continually subject to new historical and political accounts of it. Only by representing itself anew can the body reframe itself in light of these changing plots. That is, the field of having a body is not entirely delimited and stabilized as it is necessarily subject to change. It is precisely the body's potential to become a stranger to itself or a stranger to others that incentivizes us to continue representing ourselves.

The body finds its illusion of unity (belonging) when it is inscribed to the terms in which hospitality occurs; where there is a host (the other), a guest (the body) and a witness or place. These are the coordinates (or conditions) that posit the body inside language where one is named (represented). As I have discussed in this book, the name secures the narcissistic cohesion of the image of the body. The name also hosts the body during life and encompasses its relations to others. We may then say that a stranger, in the most general sense, is one whose narcissistic cohesion of the image of the body is broken or that cannot find a host or a place that recognizes them. A stranger is one whose presence is not legitimate in the domain of language.

Speaking of language as the host in the house of the body, Derrida questioned: "What in fact does language name, the so-called mother tongue, the language you carry with you, the one that also carries us from birth to death? Doesn't it figure the home that never leaves us? The proper or property, at least the fantasy of property that, as close as could be to our bodies." In this question, he is posing that language gives us a fantasy of property that accompanies us until death. As said earlier, language is that which enables the body to represent itself and as much as kinship is the symbolic host of the body.

In this text, Derrida is questioning whether language serves as a home that never leaves us. As I have interpreted, a break in the symbolic order rendered Antigone a stranger, so in effect, language may sometimes deny us hospitality. To me, our dependence on others for representation means that failures in the symbolic order and the repercussions these have in us render us vulnerable to this abandonment of language and therefore to becoming a stranger. The stranger is one whose house of language is broken. In the *Theban plays* (2003), we see that the house of Labdacus broke when the rules of kinship were broken by Oedipus' transgressions. Oedipus' parricide and incest put him in a broken kinship where Oedipus was both father and brother to his descendants. How then could Oedipus himself represent a body in a filiatory relationship that had been broken? And, most importantly, how would introducing Oedipus as a stranger in his own kinship, modify the norms and ideals of what a family is in Freud's Oedipal Plot?

To explore these questions within psychoanalysis, I will speak of the figure of Oedipus as the figure of a stranger. It is also necessary to explore why in this account of the Labdacus broken kinship, the status of being a stranger, repeated transgenerationally. In *Kinship Trouble in The Bacchae* (2016), Judith Butler showed how in *Oedipus Rex*, Oedipus did not recognize his mother or his father. Even though a drunken man had told him that he would kill his father and commit incest with his mother, Oedipus did not question if the man he killed could be his father. Later on, language revealed his real kinship when the drunken man's words reverberated in his body, and he understood that in effect he had slept with his mother and killed his father. It is only retrospectively that Oedipus knew that those were his parents, so therefore the prohibition of parricide and incest only works if we recognize kinship. Guilt emerges when such kinship is recognized. Why did Oedipus believe a stranger's pronouncement of who his kinship was?

It was only when Oedipus realized who his parents were that guilt emerged. I will now explore further the subject of guilt and its relation to Oedipus. In the previous chapter of this book *The Body and the Death Drive*, I posited that guilt is already present before the existence of the Oedipal Complex. I discussed how guilt is another manifestation of the death drive and that a need to be punished emerges from something beyond the conflict between the ego and the superego, which is established at the end of the Oedipal Complex. Guilt emerges as the residue of the death drive even before the appearance of this complex. I also explained how it is only through expelling erogenous masochism that the body as an archive may push towards representing itself. Oedipus' body was primarily that of a stranger, and that is why he could believe that the stranger's words represented his broken body. Then, the central conflict of Oedipus is not only a conflict of guilt for killing and committing incest but also a question of hospitality, of what it means to be a stranger and to be a body under a certain kinship.

Should we then reduce the origin of all guilt to the guilt of parricide and incest? To Freud, it seems that we should not. In *Civilization and Its Discontents* (1930), he questioned if the origin of guilt is more primitive than the deed that makes us feel remorse. His answer to this question was not explained in terms of the Oedipal Complex, but he said that guilt is a result of primordial ambivalence. Such ambivalence is present in the infant's relation to the breast. My assertion is that Oedipus' difficulty to see himself as the son of a mother and father (with whom he committed incest and parricide) is a re-edition of a primary inability to perceive the breast so that he could represent himself. Both in this moment of recognition of kinship and in the primary enigma, Oedipus was confronted with the theme of hospitality and guilt for the ambivalence towards the breast or his family. This moment involves questioning whom or what is that (the family or the breast) and who are we in the eyes of others. How do bodies as places host or represent strangers (the breast and the family)?

This question of hospitality is particularly acute in *Oedipus at Colonus in* the *Theban Plays* (2003). The tragedy recounts the exile of Oedipus from Thebes to Colonus, where he and his daughter were given shelter. Antigone led her blind father to Colonus; meanwhile, Polynices who had been cast out of Thebes decided to look for his father-brother Oedipus. At first, Oedipus refused to see him, but Antigone was able to convince her father. Polynices told him immediately that he had been outcast by Eteocles and because of this, was preparing to attack Thebes. This conflict between brothers was the direct result of Oedipus' curse. The part of the story that is relevant to our question is that as Oedipus walked into Colonus with Antigone, he had already committed the transgressions of parricide and incest and had lost a place to die. The only thing he desired was a place for his body to rest forever. "Who is king?" "What does it mean to be a king or a father?" were of no importance to him now. His concern was now centered primarily on where he would find hospitality. While contemplating this problem, he laid down in a grove that bore the marks of a holy ground. A citizen of Colonus approached and insisted that the place was forbidden to mortals and that Oedipus and Antigone could not be there. After that incident, the people in the city saw Oedipus as a total stranger, and he was told to leave. From this, we can see that neither in life nor death could Oedipus (as the figure of a stranger) have the symbolic permission to find a place for his body. Oedipus body was constituted as abject, the lack of permission to have a body and therefore a place posited him as a stranger who was continually transgressing rules and places.

This scene in *Oedipus in Colonus* in the *Theban Plays* (2003) is central. Antigone inherited the affliction of not having a place; of having a broken body, of being a stranger. Antigone, daughter and sister of Oedipus, inherited guilt as a consequence of being part of Oedipus' kinship. She commits suicide soon after being banished to a cave to die. The death of Antigone can be seen as a transgenerational repetition of the difficulty of having a body, and as we see in some bodies today, the image of the body finds no way to be represented. In a transgenerational transmission of his trauma, Oedipus' failure to find a place for his body was reenacted by Antigone. As Freud stated in *Beyond the Pleasure Principle* (1920) repetition compulsion is one of the only visible manifestations of the death drive; therefore I will continue to explore how the death drive is acting in Oedipus' body.

As a stranger, Oedipus could not find a place for his dismembered body as if the place he sought was a projection of an image of his broken body. Oedipus' dilemma of having no place of death is a dilemma that concerns the death that already existed within his broken body. The myth is about a man whose life supposedly entails a certain determinability until the death drive unlinks the representation of his body. We can then see a death-driven indeterminability in him that extends to his relations in kinship. Part of Oedipus' destruction is that he could no longer represent his body because the death drive unlinked the representation that constituted him as a body in a certain family order. Oedipus did not doubt the drunken stranger's narrative; it was because of his body's status as a stranger that he could ascribe to this narrative unquestioningly. Why didn't Oedipus ask the universal question of hospitality to the drunken man: who are you to make such a statement? Instead, he believed the stranger's emplotment of his body, and it entered into him as a parasite. From then on, his body was increasingly broken; he gouged his eyes out, he lost his place of burial and inherited the status of being a stranger to his descendants.

I have been referring to Oedipus as a stranger, so I will now explore what Freud said about this theme. Freud did not specifically define what it is to be a stranger, but in *Civilization and Its Discontents* (1930), he made certain assumptions of what being a stranger means to our own body and why we recognize others or make them abject. He also wrote about people who are not discriminating in whom they love. Interestingly, in this text, he posits that the highest aim of love was familial configuration, but he said that in spite of everything only a small minority find happiness along the path of love. According to his text, another form of love is found in people who displace the value of being loved with that of loving others. Such bodies do not direct their love towards a single object of affection but to all humans alike. But to Freud, such love is not the highest form of love, as a love that does not discriminate forfeits part of its value by doing an injustice to the object. By this, he meant that not all men are worthy of love. Moreover, he considered certain forms of love to be mature love, which in this text he circumscribes to relations of kinship under a heterosexual family plot or under an "inhibited aim" where the love is between friends. He stated that mature love is the relation between a man and a woman whose genital needs have led them to found a family and also the positive feelings between parents and children. Freud wanted to preserve the idea of a heterosexual family as a more mature kind of love.

In *Civilization and its Discontents* (1930) Freud considered love under those terms of kinship as something valuable that must not be thrown away without reflection. His conviction was that if one loves someone, they must be deserving of it. The conditions that make one eligible to deserve such love are that the person is similar to oneself (I can love myself in me) and that the love object appears as more perfect than oneself (I can love my ideal of myself in them). Then, following his way of thinking, we represent others as strangers when they are not similar to us, or when we are unable to see an ideal of ourselves in them. In the same text, Freud was critical of the commandment "Thou shalt love thy neighbor as thyself." To him, strangers are not only unworthy of love, but also more likely to demonstrate hostility and hatred. In his conception of civilization, humans are not gentle creatures who want to love and be loved, but aggressive beings whose drives are directed towards achieving recognition in culture.

We can see that Oedipus was not considering this distinction, that a stranger may not be worthy of our trust. Oedipus was a stranger whose drives were directed towards the recognition of his body under a particular plot. Because his necessity of recognition was so strong, he made no effort to discern whether the stranger was deserving of his trust and whether he should believe his words. What is universal in this myth is the understanding that part of our bodies is hosted and represented and another part is a stranger as it is not represented and therefore is inhospitable. This dilemma is universal because all bodies necessarily rely on the words of strangers (initially our parents or primary figures) to constitute themselves. In this sense, our bodies are always incomplete. Because of this inhospitable part of us, we look for hospitality in plots, and such plots may be dangerous and sometimes fatal as was the case with Antigone and Oedipus.

In *Antigone* in *The Theban Plays* (2003) Antigone's suicide is the most radical manifestation of being a stranger as her image of the body is broken and therefore is no longer able to host her abject part. By being buried alive in a tomb (the home of the dead), she is trapped in the status of inhospitability. That means that even in the last moments of her life she is a parasite because a body that is alive does not belong in the house of the dead. Because her body was broken, she found no symbolic construction to represent the difference between life and death and her illusion of immortality became real when she was buried alive. Then, the only alternative she had to end her existence as a parasitic stranger in the house of the death was to kill herself. Her difficulty to find a place in the world in life and death was a transgenerational inheritance from Oedipus who was both a stranger and an abject body who found no place to rest. Such transgenerational repetition is what lets us see how conflicts with the image of the body and hospitality, return from the unconscious.

Oedipus is a figure that allows us to see that we sometimes make abject what returns from the unconscious to be questioned and represented. But if we do not question who the stranger is within us, it erases the possibility of being hospitable to ourselves. This lack of acceptance of difference also makes others abject. The way psychoanalysis has thought of sexual difference has made abject those who are not men. Reinforcing the omnipotence of the body by making what is different abject may work as a primary form of differentiation. But what is made abject returns, and if we do not ask "Who are you?" it is made abject again. This is not only cruel but limits the spectrum of difference that could allow hospitality to exist for all bodies.

13

CLINICAL PRACTICE AND SOCIAL PHENOMENA

In this chapter, I will give some examples that not only subsume to the Oedipal Plot but to a symbolic realm that is not necessarily Oedipal; a plot that is already symbolic and therefore may belong to another form of emplotment that has not yet been named.

In 1914, Sigmund Freud's first grandson Ernst was born to his daughter Sophie and Max Halberstadt; the Hamburg photographer. Freud reacted immediately with joy, and sent a note to his friend Ferenczi. In *Letter from Sigmund Freud to Sándor Ferenczi, March 11* (1914) he wrote:

> Dear Friend,
> Tonight (10th to 11th) at 3 o'clock a little boy, my first grandchild! Very strange! An oldish feeling, respect for the wonders of sexuality! Sophie is very well; she even said over the telephone: "It wasn't so bad."
> Kind regards, to Frau G. Also.
> Yours,
> Freud

Ten years later in *The Dissolution of the Oedipal Complex* (1924) Freud had stated that femininity as such implies a phantasy of giving one's son to the father; this idea was symptomatic of the fall of the Pater Familias. Did little Ernst represent to Freud a restoration of such a fall, as seeing this baby allowed him to regain some sort of patriarchal power? Unfortunately, we cannot be certain of his unconscious motives, because we cannot ask Freud face to face and see what his defenses and reactions say about that. But we do know that Freud's observation of his grandson Ernst led to his refiguring of the pleasure principle and made him conceive of this pleasure being represented by a plot.

According to Adriana Prengler (2001) in 1915, Freud spent a few weeks with his daughter Sophie, Max and Ernest and the proud grandfather attentively observed the 18-month-old infant. Ernst was breastfed by Sophie, and she had a tender relationship with her son. *In Beyond the Pleasure Principle* (1920) Freud wrote that this boy had a judicious character and did not cry when his mother left for a few hours; it even seemed as if her absence was not difficult for him. Freud observed that when little Ernst played he was in the habit of throwing objects. Sometimes he would throw them around the room, other times, underneath the crib. Every object he found no matter how small would be part of this game to the extent that it was hard to retrieve all the objects he had thrown. As he played this game of expulsion, a game that in my interpretation re-edits abjection, he would proffer a prolonged sound: "o-o-o-o." His mother Sophie would say that what he meant was "fort," which means away. So, the infant would play repetitively that his objects went "away."

In Beyond the Pleasure Principle (1920) Freud interpreted this game as an act of disappearance as if he was repeating the trauma of the breast going away. During that same visit, Freud also observed Ernst playing with a wooden reel attached to a string. With great ability, he would cast the wooden piece out of his crib while holding onto the string with his other hand. As the object disappeared out of Ernst's sight, he would say "o-o-o-o" again, but as he reeled the object back into his crib, he'd say "Da!" (It's here!). The theme of this game was both appearance and disappearance, and he took pleasure in both, but what seemed to be most enjoyable to him, was when he made the object appear again.

For Freud (1920) in the same text, this was not just a game, as he believed games enact psychic mechanisms of profound density and are the enacting of a plot. His interpretation was that although Ernst accepted without protest when his mother went away, his play recreated how his mother's (breast) went away and contributed to his bodily formation. Throwing objects allowed him to reenact this scene of appearance and disappearance. Therefore, we can assume that for him such play was an act that helped to consolidate the limits of his body. By throwing things, he made abject what was difficult for him to bear and by appearing and disappearing things he learned what alterity is, that his mother was different from him. Freud pondered the nature of the pleasure that the expulsion of the object gave to Ernst. It made sense that the infant felt pleasure and would exclaim "da" when recovering the lost object, but what was the pleasure experienced in making objects go away? Sometimes when the infant played, he would throw things away without retrieving them. Freud then intuited that the repetition of this game brought pleasure beyond the laws of what he thought defined pleasure. Ernst experienced pleasure in the unpleasurable because although this reiterated play reenacted a painful loss, it contained an important difference: now he was a body with a certain agency in the plot.

As stated before in this book, at the beginning of bodily formation, the vulnerability of an infant means that it depends entirely on others. Ernst received bodily stimulation passively as does any infant at that stage. Now, with his game, his actively repeating the going away of his mother was a form of representing such a plot even though this reenactment was unpleasurable or somehow violent.

According to Freud in *Beyond the Pleasure Principle* (1920), a drive of revenge was also part of the pleasurable displeasure experienced by Ernst. As if he was saying to his mother "go away, I do not need you; I can even throw you away." His way of playing had the function of representing himself as having a body and being actively responsible for representing his mother and the world. Abjection plays a central role in Ernst's game of throwing things and is an example of how representing ourselves in culture implies the violence of making objects abject. I will now look at how plots have a role in how we represent ourselves in culture.

When Ernst said –o-o-o-o-, Sophie understood him to be saying "front." Given that Sophie's husband had gone to war, it is likely that she had mentioned the word "front" around Ernst. And if so, with what sentiment would she have said it? What enigmatic message would Sophie have communicated so that Ernst used the word "front" in his game? As time passed, the word took on new meaning. Later, Ernst would also punish his toys-objects and tell them "Go to the front." Now that Ernst was aware that his absent father had gone to the front in World War I, the word front meant something different to him.

What strikes me is Freud's interpretation that this would then, obviously, be part of an Oedipal Plot: the infant wanted to send his father to war because he wanted his mother to himself, having already experienced losing her in the absence of the breast. In this case, the "fort" game is not only about mastering the loss of mother but also about Ernst manifesting his mother's fear of losing her husband, Max. It was also a game that enacted the parricide wishes of the Oedipal tragedy. In *Beyond the Pleasure Principle* (1920) Freud referred to Ernst's way of playing as a "cultural achievement" in the sense that it demonstrated that he was already inserted in a symbolic realm that represents culture. That is, we can see that the infant now had a body as he represented it through play. He experienced loss, and he re-edited this loss within the symbolic realm of the Oedipal narrative. So this use of representation is one way he was able to transform Sophie's use of "front" and give different meanings to the word.

However, in the example of Ernst, we may see alternative ways of how emplotment occurs. So now I will go deeper, exploring how performativity transformed the meaning of the expression *fort-da* as Ernst played. Earlier we saw how this expression includes an Oedipal Scenario when it is edited retroactively. This scenario gives an emplotment to the body. Words affect bodies, words contain plots, with words we emplot our bodies and to Freud, all plots were Oedipal Plots. At first, when Ernst threw objects -o-o-o-o- meant something that was not Oedipal. I think it would be uncritical to say that the expression was pre-symbolic just because it was not Oedipal. In Freud's example, -o-o-o-o- was already a metaphor for the mother's absence and metaphors are symbolic figures of speech. Some analysts have said that a scene such as this one is pre-Oedipal but how could it be considered pre-Oedipal if -o-o-o-o- is already a metaphor? Are all symbolic plots Oedipal or can the performativity of symbols transform the plot into one that is not necessarily Oedipal? To me, what Freud is implying with the example of Ernst is that there are symbols that are not Oedipal. As I said, -o-o-o-o- already works as a metaphoric function that was more original than when it was subsumed to the Oedipal Plot.

The Oedipal Plot as an emplotment of power has formed the way in which we encounter alterity. So has the mechanism of abjection, which comes before the Oedipal in the development of the subject. In the example of Freud's grandchild Ernst, it was by expelling objects and making them abject that he formed an image of himself. It is as though the objects he threw represented his image of himself as an object that had been expelled from his mother in her absence. After all, the objects that represented his mother and his father were extensions of the image of his body. Therefore, alterity was an extension of the body that he expelled and threw away from himself.

The example of Ernst appears in the second part of *Beyond the Pleasure Principle* (1920), a text that starts with war, war neurosis and dreams of war as leading themes. In the middle of a text on violence, it occurred to Freud to speak of his grandson as if the maternal "violence" that Ernst experienced and reenacted in his game, was part of a bigger, social form of violence. Because bodies are historical archives, to me, his play was representing an epochal construction of war, not only an Oedipal Plot that speaks of a particular dynamic within the family. Go to the front, represents not only the Oedipal desire to send his father to war again but also the traumatic re-edition of what war means as a representational form.

By this, I refer to war as an emplotment, as an epochal narrative that affects the body and organizes the way in which drives work. I am not only referring to the drives of revenge directed towards his mother and father or to a plot involving them, but to war itself, as an object of representation. War as an object of representation is not partial like a breast, and it represents broader forms of destruction than the familial implications of the Oedipal Plot. Ernst sees his body in the mirror as a total object and he makes himself disappear when he says "Go to the Front." If he can see his body as a total object, and the world is an extension of the body, he is already able to represent what is beyond his father or his mother. That is, his body is a complete object already and because the world is an extension of the body, so are the images of his world. Not only are father or mother total objects, but so is the war that affects them all. With his game, he becomes an agent who plays with war as an object precisely because of its political effect on him. He plays war not only because he hears Sophie mention the word "front" with all the weight of its potential consequences for her, but because of how war affects him beyond its significance to his mother and father.

I disagree with analysts that consider that any scene that is not Oedipal is pre-Oedipal. According to Laplanche and Pontalis in *The Language of Psychoanalysis* (1998) the term "Pre-Oedipal" assumes that every pre-story or antenarrative (everything that is pre-symbolic) may only become symbolic by subsuming to the Oedipal Plot. The pre-Oedipal has been thought of as that which happens before the Oedipal stage of development, and it occurs in a relationship of one or two. This stage includes narcissistic identification, maternal dependency, and anarchic component drives that direct towards partial objects or towards aims that do not include a total object and primary processes where thing presentations prevail. Oedipal aspects arise when a relationship of three appears, and it includes paternal identification and competition, and specific drives and aim. In this stage, phallic erotogenicism and word presentations prevail. The Oedipal Plot is the only symbolic instance or narrative of the body used in psychoanalysis because it has been the prevailing plot in a historical context. So, the difference between pre-Oedipal and Oedipal is thought to be that the former is considered pre-symbolic and the Oedipal is when aspects arise that are symbolic forms of being inscribed in the world. In this way of thinking, culture exists only because of this specific symbolic inscription. But the example of Ernst shows us how war is a symbolic representation that exceeds the Oedipal Plot. This example shows us how a symbolic relationship with culture exists parallel to the Oedipal.

If an analysand were to speak of childhood games similar to Ernst's, one interpretation or question that would be important to ask is what war means to them. Then to explore what kind of traumatic impressions are being repeated in such a narrative and in the relationship with the analyst. The analyst needs to value this narrative as something of no lesser value than what is Oedipal. It is important to observe what role abjection has in this kind of play, and recognize how this game of throwing objects reiterates making the analysand and their objects abject, including the analytic relationship. Reiteration that speaks of abjection needs to be interpreted, as making others abject is at the core of how the body rigidly represents itself. Such an interpretation might offer other possibilities for them to represent their body and alterity.

Ernst's games were not only a symbolic feature that spoke metaphorically of his relationship with his parents but also in a parallel form were representing his body in a political context. His body was being represented as a total object and simultaneously as a political archive in an emplotment of war which exceeded the narrative of the familial Oedipal Plot. The emplotment of war acted upon Ernst, it marked his body and affected the way he related to his objects and the world; but not only that, it shaped the very process by which Ernst formed an image of himself and others. If as analysts we interpret only the dynamic within the family configuration, a rigid image of the body is reinforced. But if, as is done here, the analyst questions the other possible meanings of war it allows the body of the patient to represent a more dynamic image of his body. In this example, Ernst's play transformed the meaning of the expression Fort-Da. If we were to interpret such an image strictly under the Oedipal Plot, the image of the body would become rigid but if we stay with the dynamicity of the image of his body by asking him what war means, new forms of emplotment might occur. In this specific case, resignifying war is of primal importance. Asking questions related to the objects that the patient is struggling to represent could open a space for them to signify what is being made abject and imagine a different future of alterity that is not only constructed through abjection.

Although Freud did not receive infants as patients, he did listen to what their parents said about them and took a special interest in childhood play that involved expulsion. In both the case of artist Goethe in *A Childhood Recollection from "Dichtung Und Wahrheit"* (1917) and the clinical case of The Rat Man in *Notes upon a*

Case of Obsessional Neurosis (1909), they remembered themselves throwing things away when they were little just like Ernst did. This, Freud interpreted as a symbolic action of throwing away their younger brothers. Their brothers represented a threat to the imagined preference that their mothers had for them. To him, this game of expulsion was a re-edition of the Oedipal familial configuration.

It is clear that in the cases Freud mentioned, there is an Oedipal content in the game of throwing objects; however, it is evident to me that there is something more than the Oedipal Plot involved in this play. Freud's mandate of the Oedipal as the angular stone of psychoanalysis has made it difficult for an analyst to think of symbolic narratives that do not necessarily ascribe to the Oedipal Plot. In the perspective of some contemporary analysts, most patients operate in a pre-symbolic realm just because their narratives do not belong to the Oedipal Plot. If as analysts we want to alleviate the suffering of today's bodies, in our practice we must struggle to listen to narratives that escape an adscription within the Oedipal Plot in spite of the weight of the angular stone.

I will now speak of examples from my clinical practice and from cultural phenomena where something more than Oedipal is evident in today's emplotments of the body.

*****

A 20-year-old artist from Argentina who was living in Mexico City called my office to get a first appointment. When I asked for her name, she seemed to have difficulty answering but then said in a louder voice "my name is Ale … x … Alexandra!." This hesitancy, as to whether she wanted me to call her Alexandra, Ale or Alex, reflected her trouble delimiting her identity. During her first sessions with me, she elaborated that each of those names had a different use. She preferred to be called Alexandra by the people that held her in esteem. Ale was the name she used at the lesbian bars when she was looking to meet other women. Alex was the name she most liked, and it was the name she used especially for social media; her ex-boyfriends called her Alex. This difficulty to give her name was very telling for what developed afterward during analysis.

Her father was a very important businessman with a perverse profile who after receiving death threats had hired a clandestine service to intercept the telephone lines of all the members of his family. She told me that she was aware that her father spied on her cell phone and that he also sent bodyguards to follow her everywhere. Although she recognized that it was not normal, she excused her father's behavior as neurotic subjects do within an Oedipal configuration. Everything she spoke of in these first sessions had a strong impact on my body as a listener, but she seemed to be numb to these experiences. As she narrated these events, her body gestures were undynamic, and when I pointed this out to her, she said that she had felt that way for a long time. She told me that sometimes her body felt frozen and she was unable to react. Soon after, she remembered that ten years ago, when a friend of her father attempted to have sex with her, she was unable to do anything to stop him. Every day, although her father was in the room next door, his friend would enter her room and sexually abuse her. As she recounted this she laughed and said how crazy it sounded. When I asked about what was going on with her as she spoke of this, she became frozen again. Thinking within the Oedipal Plot, I questioned how if she were a hysterical subject this would be a phantasy of abuse and her bodily reactions would be a representation of an Oedipal Plot wherein the primary scene she is with a man and her father sees her. But added to this emplotment within the Oedipal Scenario, in countertransference I felt her anger, her numbness and the deep sense of fear she held.

Following the Oedipal interpretation I asked her how could her father not have noticed that his friend was abusing her when he kept track of every movement she made and spied on her phone. When I pointed out how scary that scenario sounded, her body shook, she cried, got up out of her seat, and started pacing. "I don't know! This is so strange!" Something happened with the Oedipal interpretation that mobilized her body from being frozen to being active. But at the same time, the dynamic image of the body that would allow her to move would now represent something other than the Oedipal Plot. "I don't know! This is so strange!" was speaking of another emplotment, one that she was afraid to think of. As that session was coming to an end, I returned to her name, by saying: "It's time, this is the end of today's session Alexandra Gonzáles."

As I have discussed in this book, the name secures the narcissistic cohesion of the image of the body. The name also hosts the body during life and encompasses its relations to others. My return to Alejandra's name was to host her particular forms of abjection, her narcissistic bond that was broken and split into many names. As I explained earlier, a stranger, in the most general sense, is one whose narcissistic cohesion of the image of the body is broken, one who cannot find hospitality or a place that recognizes them. Session after session Alexandra would doubt whether she should stay in treatment or not and constantly provoked me so that I would tell her to go away. She had become a stranger in a radical way; by way of transference, her struggle to be present in my office reflected her struggle to be hosted in the domain of language, to live within her own name.

At a certain point, Alejandra told me that her father had intercepted my cell phone and sometimes sent his bodyguards to spy on me. Information that she knew about me seemed to confirm that this was true. The situation was something I found terrifying, and it was the subject of many hours of therapy with my analyst. I also discussed this patient with my supervisor; some days we would elucidate her neurotic, psychotic and perverse defenses to the primary scene in the Oedipal Scenario. What was frequently seen was a dislocation, a psychosomatic break between soma and body that made it difficult for her to give a symbolic account of her body under her name. In one group supervision, some of my colleagues suggested that her case was not Oedipal and that she should be in another kind of treatment. Others commented that patients with this kind of problematic usually discontinue therapy. What to me is indisputable is that this case points to a crisis in listening for analysts; a crisis that speaks of an epistemic crisis of the body that needs to be addressed. As analysts, we are responsible for listening to and responding to this crisis in a way that does not make certain bodies abject. We must struggle to think of alternate emplotments as Freud did when he found an emplotment for the bodies of his time.

As I continued to interpret this patient's defenses, I observed how her interaction with me mirrored her relationship with objects. Our sessions focused on integrating the three different images that formed her way of seeing herself, and I listened for the emplotments she embodied. She began to stay longer than the allotted time, and the sessions were always difficult. Her erotic transference increased considerably; I think this was not only a strategy to stop working with me, but was also a struggle to give her disperse libidinal forces a unity of object. As these forces gained unity, a new emplotment emerged. She started to have doubts about the effect that using so many names had on her, wondering if maybe it had prevented her from assuming only one sexed position, one identity. One day, she told me that she wanted to be on her own for a while and that she would be going back to Argentina. In our last session, I explained what we had been working on and that sometimes it felt like she needed time to figure out her body image. The sessions that worked on her incapacity to represent her difficult experiences and to host herself under one name had a mobilizing effect, and in time something beyond the incestuous plot emerged.

Months later, this patient wrote to me: "I have seen an analyst called Fernando and will be continuing to work with him. My life is calm, and I am grateful to you for that. I have now assumed the name Alexandro and will be undergoing hormonal treatment to become a man." Alexandro also wrote that he thought that he was ready to fall in love and that his art projects would now be destined to explore ways that human relationships can be less violent and also to defend the rights of transexuals. Alejandro has chosen a name for himself and a symbolic emplotment of the body that does not correspond to the Oedipal Plot. His letter describes a plot that is not Oedipal, but it is symbolic. Then, could we really say that because the plot is not Oedipal, it is necessarily pre-Oedipal? Or, as seen in the case of Ernst where he was representing an epochal construction of war that was difficult to think about, is there another plot being represented by Alexandro that is already symbolic but that it is difficult for us to think of as well? Especially if we consider that assuming a sexed position is a mark of having assumed a symbolic place in culture. Assuming his sex, imagining he might fall in love soon and finding a way in which he may defend the rights not only of himself but also of others, are ways that this patient is exploring to host alterity. Alterity allows relationships that are not pre-Oedipal, and in this example, we can see clearly how his way of emploting difference exceeds the idea of difference that was stated by Freud within the Oedipal Plot.

What symbolic narrative is contained in the plots of patients like this one whose image of the body is not Oedipal? We as analysts have to be open to listening for other forms of symbolic content as often our listening is impeded by Freud's Oedipal Shibboleth. If reading this narrative was disturbing for you, you would do well to question how much of that is due to abjection. Do you think it would have been better for me to have said, "I cannot take your case"; in other words, I will not listen to you? Hospitality requires bravery and the willingness to sustain communication with the other. That is what Freud taught by example when he treated hysterical patients and actively listened to the unconscious plot behind their behavior.

★★★★

Recently I was scrolling down my Facebook timeline and saw a post by the BBC titled *Sophia the Robot Wants a Baby and Says Family is Really Important* (2017). The post was about Sophia, a female robot that was created in Hong Kong using breakthrough robotics and artificial intelligence technology. I read that amid much controversy, the robot was granted citizenship in Saudi Arabia. This robot is not required to wear the headscarf and abaya, nor the burka that is customary there. Given that women are still in a position of subordination and are made abject, how does it affect the bodies of women that a female robot is given citizenship, an ID, and other rights that women of that same country do not share? Do new technologies such as this one reinforce the abjection of women?

The current epistemic crisis of the body involves a difficulty in assimilating: we are living under the confluence of an Oedipal Plot and of other plots that have not yet been named. This confluence confronts us with a transformation of the concept of the body. Because of this, we need to struggle to find a metaphor for the bodies of our time. How will we give an account of the bodies of our time if we do not listen to the emplotments they are manifesting as Freud did when he gave a metaphoric account of the bodies of his day? What bodies experience today is not the same as what was happening in Freud's time. Technology has changed the limits of our bodies. Cellphones have become extensions of ourselves; if I am in the middle of a conversation and have a doubt, I can Google information on my phone. With a touch of a screen, my knowledge is expanded as if the screen were an addition to my memory. Another example of this is how the father of my patient figuratively controlled the mobility of Alejandro's body by spying on his cellphone.

Technology has changed the concept of our body and its limitations. Transplants make it possible to prolong our lives; plastic surgery and sex reassignment surgery have changed the limits of what is possible for our bodies. The existence of these surgeries grants different possibilities within the symbolic laws of our bodies and to our sexed positions. New weapons technologies such as bombs, chemical weapons and drones have also made possible different forms of violence. Whereas before, killing required a physical encounter of bodies, these weapons allow bodies to inflict damage without being physically present. A shocking example of this is how it is now possible to send a small drone into a house and silently kill the designated individual(s) without anyone noticing. The concept of alterity changes when there is no physical encounter. This technology allows a virtual physicality, the drone an extension of the body of the killer. The bodily extension travels to where it kills its target, requiring no physical encounter between the victim and the sender. The drone can then pulverize the murdered body, its disappearance so complete that the body is ungrievable as one cannot represent a body without knowing if that body was killed or not. Not only is technology contributing to an epistemic crisis of the body, but also to the ways alterity is thought of, in the sense that these technologies may contribute to a lack of accountability.

Technology has also given us new options for reproduction which in turn are making new forms of kinship possible. The advent of contraception means that sexual relations are no longer necessarily linked to having children or having a family. Techniques of assisted reproduction have meant that a heterosexual couple is not necessary to have a family. Because of these technologies, families conformed by same-sex couples may have biological children and create a form of kinship that does not necessarily ascribe to the classic familial configuration of the Oedipal Plot. Additionally, the option of renting a womb creates very different dynamics than that of the Oedipal scene. Also, genetic technology allows us to intervene in the physicality of the body of the fetus so that the conscious desires of the parents can now have a factual impact on the somatic body of this new life.

What crisis are these technologies producing in the epistemic body? What new emplotments of the body will encompass the changes that technology offers? The place that men held in the family plot has been forever changed by these techniques of reproduction. As studied before in this book, before modernity, God and men were considered to be the creators of life. In the last century, an epistemic crisis emerged with the fall of god and the acceptance of the idea that recognized the uterus as property of women. Now, with donated sperm, a woman and technology can produce children. There is, however, a certain irony in the fact that women may now have a baby through technology, but a robot in Saudi Arabia is afforded more rights than the women of that country. It would seem that technology responds to a plot where women continue to be made abject.

There are many examples of how women are being made abject by the gender violence inflicted by the Oedipal patriarchal plot. By making women abject, the Oedipal Complex confers normality to this violence. Gender violence is pervasive everywhere, as the recent #MeToo movement has evidenced. According to Nadia Khomami, in *#MeToo: How a hashtag became a rallying cry against sexual harassment* (2017), this movement has gained momentum in the US and has become a rallying cry against sexual harassment and the erasure of women's voices. Within 24 hours, 4.7 million people around the world engaged in the #MeToo conversation, with over 12m posts, comments and reactions. Silence has been complicit in femicides and is this also a factor in the gender violence being denounced by the #MeToo movement. Only because of the willingness of all those women to speak out could the widespread incidence of abuse be exposed, and we owe to feminism for this possibility. Bodies that lack visibility in today's heteropatriarchal society are invisible because they are made abject by the society whose death drive posits them as unrepresentable. This is why it is urgent that we continue to speak up about gender violence and any other way in which women or any gender representing feminine attributes are made abject.

The statistics I will now present are from Mexico because I think it is significant that although this country has one of the highest rates of femicides, few people are protesting this reality. In Mexico, these crimes are significantly underreported. Available statistics only quantify the reporting of these crimes but will never account for the pain of these women nor are representative of the actual prevalence of gender violence. According to INMUJERES (2016) every day, seven femicides are reported in Mexico; according to the Mexican Government, women in this country between the ages of 15 to 45 years old are more likely to be killed or assassinated than to contract HIV or to get cancer. Female political candidates in the states of Chiapas, Puebla, Tabasco, and Tlaxcala are continually subject to death threats. The United Nations declared that every four minutes a rape occurs in this country and 63 percent of 15-year-old women had experienced gender violence. It is estimated that over 40 percent of the population of women have been sexually abused. Just in March 2017, 1219 rapes were reported. Seventy percent of these violations occur within the family context. Authorities have said that 38 percent of rapes are not reported; however, it is likely that this percentage is even higher.

In September 2017, a month before the #MeToo movement gained momentum; a march took place in Mexico City to protest the high rate of femicides in the country and women's issues in general. The march was also calling for justice to be imparted in recent incidents of violence against women that had met with impunity. One of the groups that participated was a small collective of women who were denouncing the unequal state of privilege between men and women. Newspaper *Sin Embargo* (2017) said that when eight men including journalist Jenaro Villamil attempted to join them they were asked by the women to please walk with another group as walking together as women was an important part of the statement they were trying to make. The men not only ignored their petition, but they walked in front of the collective acting as though they were leading the group. The women again asked them to leave, but they refused to and instead called the women's request sexist. The cynicism displayed by these men is impressive; in this example, the reiterative force of misogyny and the current backlash against progress in women's issues is evident.

In this chapter, I give examples of symbolic emplotments that are not necessarily Oedipal. The example of Ernst's throwing objects is an account of how Freud had considered this game to be a performance of psychic mechanisms of profound density that represented the pleasurable displeasure of re-experiencing how his parents (objects) left. I argue that with this game, he was not only enacting the Oedipal familial configuration, but it also represented an emplotment of war. My critique of the use of the term pre-Oedipal to denominate all that is pre-symbolic is founded on the observation that there are symbolic emplotments that are not Oedipal and that do not seek to become Oedipal in the future either.

In the clinical case of Alexandra, we can see that the relationship with her father was incestuous in the sense that he almost certainly knew that his friend was abusing her. Within the Oedipal Plot, her body was paralyzed in a hysterical conversion where her body spoke of a phantasy of incest. Outside of the Oedipal Plot, her body was paralyzed in a psychosomatic break as she could no longer bear this emplotment. I explain how this traumatic experience broke her image of the body so that she became a stranger in the house of language and could not find hospitality within her own name. Her letter shows how the pre-symbolic configuration that had impeded her achieving narcissistic unity became symbolic afterward in an emplotment that was not Oedipal.

This patient's story exemplifies how women continue to be carriers of abjection in our culture; that which represents feminine attributes is still being made abject. Alexandra's father as an accomplice of her abuse is symptomatic of this cultural problem. To give another example of the abjection of women in the cultural domain, I speak of how the #MeToo movement has brought the issue of gender violence into the public spotlight. This movement is proving to be an effective tool to break the silence around this topic, which historically has been complicit in the perpetration of abjection. I also mention the case of the robot Sophia that has been granted more sovereignty than the women of her country and how this reproduces the traditional emplotment of patriarchy but at the same time presents a new emplotment of the body where technology changes the episteme of the body. This chapter also discusses how new technologies make it possible to enact violence or reproduce life without physical contact between bodies and that this is changing the emplotments available today.

The current epistemic crisis of the body makes it evident that to deal with alterity in a responsible way we need to have a genuine encounter with it. The difficulty that some bodies are having today to find a symbolic emplotment is breaking the image of these bodies. A broken image of the body is a broken image of others, and I believe this crisis asks us to revise how we deal with alterity. I am not stating that we need to protect ourselves from the new technologies or the epistemic crisis, but that we need to take responsibility for the changes they bring. This is why throughout this book I sustain that if we are to find a future for alterity, we will need to think of possible emplotments of the body that are not necessarily Oedipal. A seminal drift of the meanings of the Oedipal sign is necessary, so that the sign may include new forms of understanding difference.

CONCLUSIONS

This work has focused on two specific concepts: the body and the Oedipal Complex as an emplotment of the body. I began by using Preciado's definition of the body in *Inappropriate Bodies* (2014) and in *Somatheque* (2012) as a somatic-psychic archive that store political and social practices in it and used it as a lens to read Freudian theory. Then stated how, to become a body, we necessarily ascribe to emplotments that allow us to belong to culture. Also discussed, was how the meanings and significance that we attach to our materiality to become bodies as archives, do not float free of that materiality.

My critical reading of the Oedipal Complex considers the difficulties Freud's Oedipal Plot presents to the bodies of today. I describe how Freud observed bodies that were undergoing an epistemic crisis and how his Oedipal Plot offered an emplotment to symbolize those bodies. Taking into account Preciado's notion of epistemic crisis of the body in *Inappropriate Bodies* (2014) the subject of hysteria was revised, revealing how these patient's symptoms were the manifestations of a modern political fiction of the body. According to Preciado (2014) before the 18th century, the uterus was represented as a floating base in a vacuous space that belonged to the Pater Familias. Reproduction was believed to take place in the drop of the sperm and not within the body. This meant that bodies were thought to be a creation of men and God and ontologically women's bodies were a failure. The Word of God as the symbolic instance that sustained women's uteri fell as God fell and the idea of the uterus belonging to women emerged. Women's bodies were confronted with that epistemic crisis and they would have to appropriate a body that had not been considered to be their own.

To me, the manifestations of hysterical bodies expressed the difficulty women had to appropriate their body. As the Pater Familias fell, bodies struggled to find a new plot different from the Word of God that would represent them. Inspired by Dolto (1984) I defended that when bodies do not find a symbolic order that will represent them, the limits of the body become blurry and the unity of the body breaks. Freud's exceptional intellect conceived of an emplotment that would give a certain order to those broken bodies. The cultural references archived in Freud's body inspired his elaboration of the Oedipal Complex. This Complex placed a tragedy in the center of the formation of the body and gave an account of the drives and mechanisms that configured the bodies he observed. In psychoanalysis, the Oedipal Plot is the main representative of the drives and it became the unconscious plot with which a psychoanalyst interprets. Freud stated in *Three Essays on the theory of Sexuality* (1905) that the Oedipal Complex was the shibboleth of psychoanalysis and he went even further to say that those who do not ascribe to the concept could not call themselves psychoanalysts. So then, we can see that the bodies of analysts are doubly affected by this concept: in one dimension, because of the way our body ascribes culturally to the sign of Oedipus, in another, because it dictates our way of listening to patients. Although I praise what Freud envisioned in his time, bodies are subject to historical change, to different plots and the use of the Oedipal Plot as the only emplotment that forms bodies makes many of today's bodies abject.

Before presenting my conclusion, I will summarize what each part of the book addressed. Part I endeavors to explain what the concept of a body is within psychoanalytic theory. First, I presented Freud's perspective on the body taken from his complete works and then Laplanche, Bick, Dolto, Piera Aulagnier, Joyce McDougall and Wollheim's works were discussed to further explore the image of the body and the body-ego. It was especially important to explain what the term body is referring to, because in psychoanalysis today there is a lack of consensus and clarity regarding the concept of body, and this has been a problem for the psychoanalytic field. Recently conferences have centered the body as the main topic, but the concept of the body was almost never discussed. It is urgent to address this issue because a psychoanalyst by definition listens to bodies and interprets them. Defining what a body is, is central. Without a clear definition of the body, how can an analyst think of the subject who is asking for their help?

As I examined through this book, Freudian theory states that one is not born with a body, but it is continually formed by the act of representing. In psychoanalysis, the body is a somatic-psychic archive of memories that is not equivalent to the anatomic body. The body is incomplete as it is always longing for a reality beyond that which is circumscribed by its biology. It is the primary caregiver who transmits to the infant the experience of its body being something different from the world. This experience is first represented by the mother, through her desires and her way of being immersed in the world. A body is an archive that absorbs a set of cultural codes via its caregiver. It is a body that comes into existence by way of word-representation. The infant's psychic value emerges as a body that can represent and therefore to phantasize using a language it has imbibed. Through phantasy, a psychic operation of a symbolic nature occurs and places the body in a position of subjectivity in relation to the bodies of others. Because of the existence of phantasy, the world as we represent it is a projection of the body as an archive, of our subjectivities. Plots form bodies but also the existence of these plots depends on bodies enacting their narratives. This reliance on plots to continue to form itself makes the body vulnerable and dependent. Its vulnerability before others is the very condition for a body to represent itself. The body affirms its own existence as a negative imprint of the existence of others. While at the same time, otherness circumscribes the body in a set of cultural codes. That is, a voice lives within us that is foreign to our consciousness, it is the voice of a stranger and the narrator of our unconscious plots.

To become bodies, we are necessarily alienated in the words of others, and at the same time, something within our body resists absolute representation so our body can keep on representing itself. This alienation means that within our bodies there is always a status of being foreign, of being a stranger. The body is inevitably broken, a body divided between what it can represent and what is still unrepresentable: a division that proves to be the very condition of its representation. The unconscious appears because the body is broken. The body cannot be entirely realized, as it is in a constant process of representation, in communication with others and vulnerable to transformation by the return of the unconscious. The body as representation is always vulnerable to psychosomatic breakdown; one has a body, but that body has places where it is fractured, damaged, defective, fragmented, mutilated. In other words, the body is incomplete, its unity illusory. Of course, the body is a necessary illusion for otherness and difference to exist.

What captivated me in the process of writing this book is how the existence of difference depends on the very plots that the body uses to represent itself. I also became interested in how some plots circumscribe bodies in such a rigid way that these bodies are unable to represent other forms of existence and, therefore, make other bodies abject in radically violent ways. This led me to question the consequences of the Oedipal Plot and to question what can be done with this plot to avoid thinking of difference in terms of abjection. As I said, the body is vulnerable to plots, and the Oedipal Plot has become the predominant plot that circumscribes bodies. When this plot makes bodies abject it banishes them to the domain of the unintelligible, ignoring what their bodies are announcing. Our incapacity to consider alternative plots to represent the bodies of today, speaks of (the existence of) a deathly rigidity in the cultural domain and the difficulty we are having to give an account of a difference beyond abjection.

One part of this book uses Kristeva's concept of abjection in *Powers of Horror* (1982) and Judith Butler's notion of abject bodies in *Bodies that Matter* (1993) as a main point. Although I only mention it once, this idea is central to my thesis. Butler (1993) states that abjection is crucial to the formation of the body; the body affirms itself by expelling what it thinks it is not. This process forms the first boundaries of the body that limit what is internal and external; what is to be included and what is to be excluded from the domain of intelligibility. Abject bodies are those who are made unintelligible by an exclusionary matrix.

Then, we can say that the Oedipal Plot is a narrative that circumscribes some bodies within a category of privilege and makes others abject. As they are part of an unintelligible domain, abject bodies may ascribe to other plots that have not yet been thought of. For psychoanalysis to listen to all bodies, it is necessary to think of such plots, as Preciado (2014) and Roudinesco (2015) propose, and to question what can be done in psychoanalysis with the Oedipal Plot as it excludes certain bodies. With several levels of argumentation, I explained that the Oedipal Complex does not give an account of all bodies today and that this shibboleth of psychoanalysis is an exclusionary matrix. However, as the very condition for a body to form is the force of abjection, any plot by definition works as an exclusionary matrix of bodies. This is why I posit that for abjection to be thinkable the question of what it is to be a stranger must be placed in the center of the Oedipal Plot. Only if a plot allows bodies to be aware of how what the body makes abject is present within the unconscious, will an effort be made to elaborate what has been relegated as unintelligible in these bodies.

Bodies are subject to historical emplotments, and the Oedipal Plot is an account of the problematics of a modern epistemic crisis of the body. Today many bodies still ascribe to the Oedipal Plot; however, other bodies present new crisis because the limits of what is possible for the body have changed. Reproduction is now possible in ways that do not ascribe to heterosexual practices, bodies can be changed through cosmetic surgery, and different technologies have altered the way we relate to each other. Therefore, the domain of what may be thinkable has also changed.

I explained how in psychoanalysis the Oedipal Complex has worked as a specific emplotment that has generated an exclusionary matrix not only for the body but also for the way the analyst listens to what a body is. This exclusionary matrix has created a problem that is urgent to address, which is of thinking that a body that does not correspond to certain forms of the Oedipal Complex is necessarily pre-oedipal, perverse, psychotic or even "unthinkable." The work of psychoanalysis needs to stop making abject what does not correspond to a restrictive plot of normality and struggle towards thinking of that which causes suffering and what that suffering is announcing. This is why the task of analytic listening needs to incorporate an assimilation of difference that exceeds the exclusionary limits of abjection.

Psychoanalytic theory states that listening is done case by case as every patient has an individual way of suffering and that we should listen without memory or desire. This, in practice, is illusory as our bodies as psychoanalysts are crossed by Oedipal constructions and theories of Oedipus. The Oedipal Plot circumscribes the body of the analyst to a certain way of listening within the Oedipal Plot. This plot determines what sexual difference means and it outlines incest and parricide as the main prohibitions and desires to interpret. Moreover, the analyst determines the structure of the body of the analyzand depending on the mechanism used in response to the primal scene of the Oedipal Plot: repression, disavowal or repudiation. But, as I have said, the Oedipal Plot is a historical account, and other emplotments of the body may be determining the formation of those bodies that do not correspond to it.

It is entirely different to say that a body does not correspond to the Oedipal Plot and therefore it is unthinkable than to say that we fail to listen to some bodies because we have been too attached to the Oedipal Plot and therefore we make other forms of being abject. Because in the first option the analyst through abjection would be killing the otherness of the patient, it gives free rein to the murderous and incestuous desires of the analyst that the Oedipal Plot is supposed to regulate. The second option allows us to keep on thinking of what a body is beyond abjection. In the middle of today's epistemic crisis of the body, it is necessary that analysts stand up for what is made abject.

One way to curb such violent abjection would be to stop placing the Oedipal Complex as central to psychoanalysis. Elisabeth Roudinesco (2015) and Paul Preciado (2014) have suggested the removal of this exclusionary matrix and the creation of new myths to take its place. Although I definitely agree with their premise, I think something supplementary to the creation of new myths is needed. Oedipus as a linguistic sign has been thought of in a very specific way within psychoanalytic theory and as a sign has already had an impact in the formation of bodies. Therefore, substitution of the myth would involve more than just eradicating the concept. Through this book, I have been presenting how the Oedipal Plot has been an agent in the creation of bodies. If we were only to replace the myth with another myth, it would not change the effects that Oedipus as a linguistic sign has already had on bodies. I think that our agent (Oedipus as a sign) must not be eliminated because its elimination would augur its return. It is imperative that psychoanalytic theory restate what otherness means. This would expand the limits under which a body may be representable and give the symbolic coordinates within theory to understand difference beyond abjection. Therefore, what this book proposes is working with the iterability of the sign Oedipus within psychoanalytic theory. To do this, I worked with Oedipus in Colonus to expand the meaning of the Oedipal Plot. I concentrated on what this narrative says about otherness and about what it means to be a stranger so as to evidence Oedipus' failure of representation, Oedipus´ abjection. His status as a stranger places such failure as universal and denounces that the Oedipal Complex does not allow us to think of difference beyond abjection.

This book argues that thinking of Oedipus beyond the Oedipal Plot necessarily changes the status of unrepresentability of abject bodies. By this, I mean that if Oedipus is identified as a stranger, the Oedipal Plot changes to allow what has been made abject to be represented. We know that the very condition for becoming a body is abjection, but as I advanced in this investigation, I came to see that difference may be understood in terms that go beyond the limits of abjection.

In the second part of the book, I recounted the effect being organized under the Oedipal Plot has had on the concept of difference in psychoanalysis. Then, I wrote of Oedipus as a stranger to dislocate the matrix under which some bodies have an absolute status of representability (men) and others do not. The dislocation of this matrix would necessarily change the status of irrepresentability of abject bodies. However, even those Oedipal subjects who are under the matrix of intelligibility are still subject to being strangers; therefore, no one has absolute status of representability.

As Laplanche and Pontalis condensed in *Life and Death in Psychoanalysis* (1985), the Oedipal Complex is the organized group of ambivalent desires (love and aggression) that the infant experiments regarding its caregivers during the phallic stage (3–5 years old). The complex also presents itself in adult life when desiring the death of a rival and with sexual desire towards the opposite sex. The dissolution of the Oedipal Complex is silent during the latency period and is relived during puberty. Sexuality re-edits in the Oedipal Complex and ends by circumscribing the body under the Oedipal Plot.

According to Freud in *The Infantile Genital Organization* (1923), noticing sexual difference happens in the Oedipal Complex in the middle of a primal scene where children see the body of a person of a sex that does not correspond to the same sex as the child's body. To him, all children have sexual theories where they attribute a penis to all human beings so that difference between the sexes can only be understood in terms of a castration. The boy's estimate of the value of the penis as the universal and essential constituent in the domain of the intelligible relies on his inability to imagine a person similar to him without a penis. Then, the idea of difference for Freud relies on one particular sexual organ to represent it, an organ that only men have. Consequently, sexual difference in psychoanalysis erases any category of difference that is not explained by the penis as a representative.

In the book, I pointed out how Freud understood in *The Dissolution of the Oedipal Complex* (1924) feminine bodies as those who desire something that men have (the phallus) which in an equation transposes into having a baby as a symbolic gift for her father. Then, femininity, as conceived of by Freud belonged to a sense of property, to the terrain of the Pater Familias. This posits femininity in a very particular kinship where a woman offers her body to create life and give it to her father. Men, on the other hand, repress the incestuous and murderous desires entirely in order to leave their family and love a new one. I posed that Freud's notion of femininity was an attempt to repair the fall of the Pater Familias by desiring to give the father a baby precisely because the Pater Familias was lacking power to give life.

An emplotment that circumscribes all bodies in the domain of intelligibility and anything else in the domain of unintelligibility is very different from a plot where only men are circumscribed to the domain of what is not to be made abject. The Oedipal Plot is a narrative that posits heterosexual masculinity in the domain of intelligibility and any other sexual difference in the domain of what is unthinkable. This is why I stated that other plots are needed to represent those bodies who have been made unintelligible in the cultural domain and that return from the unconscious. If we believe that all bodies may be circumscribed in the domain of the intelligible, even though there will always be failures of representation, we would need to implement other ways of understanding difference, ones that will not make some humans abject.

In this book, I have argued that thinking of Oedipus beyond the Oedipal Plot changes the status of unrepresentability of abject bodies within the psychoanalytic domain. To change this status of abject bodies, I propose that we think of Oedipus as one who suffered from unrepresentability. This strategy does not invent new plots, but exposes the limits of the Oedipal Plot and reveals how the abjection of other bodies is a mere projection of the broken image of the body. Thinking beyond the Oedipal Plot requires that we confront the present rigidity of the image of the Oedipal body that determines what is representable and makes other plots and forms of being abject.

I introduced the idea of Oedipus as the figure of a stranger. A stranger is one whose narcissistic cohesion of the image of the body is broken; one who finds no symbolic host or place to be inscribed in. In *Oedipus in Colonus* in the *Theban Plays* (ed. 2003), Antigone leads Oedipus who was now blind into the city. He had already committed parricide and incest, had gouged his eyes out and now only wished for a place to rest forever. Oedipus was no longer asking himself who is king, or what does it mean to be a king or a father? He was more concerned with where he would find hospitality. At this point in the story, Oedipus was a stranger whose presence was not legitimate under the house of language. If there is something universal in the tragedy of Oedipus, it is his status as a stranger; it is universal in the sense that all bodies are vulnerable to breakability because as we depend on plots to represent ourselves, this status of being a stranger is within each of us.

Oedipus' place in kinship was lost because of his transgressions and that left him without a place of burial. Later in Colonus, when Oedipus transgressed their holy space, the people of the city saw him as a stranger and asked him to leave. Again, not only did he lose an appropriate physical resting place for his body, but he also lost the symbolic coordinates that assign a position of belonging. As a consequence of Oedipus' dislocation in kinship, Antigone not only inherited guilt, but also the affliction of not having a place, of having a broken body and being a stranger. Eventually, she committed suicide. Her death can be seen as a transgenerational re-edition of the difficulty of having a body. As with some bodies today, the image of her body found no way to be represented.

Oedipus' broken body left him a stranger to himself. This was why he accepted the words of the drunken stranger without questioning them. He then made an emplotment for his body out of those words. This emplotment had a profound effect on his body configuration and his place in kinship. The Labdacus' status as strangers confronts us with that which is a stranger in us. This status as a stranger is universal, but it manifests in more powerful forms if one is made abject. Denying this part of us that is a stranger, erases difference and posits the stranger as an abject body. Not asking ourselves who we are and who the other is makes us or those others parasites. This failure to understand difference beyond abjection happens when the death drive takes over the body to unlink the representations that allow us to see others as intelligible. Understanding of difference occurs when with the help of the drives of life, we represent what is different in others as singular and valuable. This way of going beyond abjection enables us to keep on representing.

Reinforcing the omnipotence of the body by making what is different abject, may work as a primary form of differentiation. But what is made abject sometimes returns from the unconscious, and making it abject again instead of asking "who are you?" deprives us of the opportunity to develop another way of understanding difference in which hospitality may be given to others and to ourselves. Oedipus is the figure that allows us to see that what returns from the unconscious needs to be questioned and represented, not to do so puts our life at risk and the lives of others. Through plots, we represent ourselves and try to quell the terrible confusion caused by the broken status of our bodies. As we can see with the Oedipal Plot, plots stop working when the narrative erases the prohibition to kill and to commit incest. That failure enhances the omnipotence of some bodies and reinforces the abjection of others. It is necessary to doubt any emplotment that entraps bodies in a rigidly normative system, precisely because these plots promote a more radical erasure of alterity.

BIBLIOGRAPHY

Anon (2017). Sophia the Robot Wants a Baby and Says Family is Really Important. BBC. Retrieved from www.bbc.co.uk/newsbeat/article/42122742/sophia-the-robot-wants-a-baby-and-says-family-is-really-important.

Anon (2017). El periodista Jenaro Villamil es sacado de la marcha de mujeres en la Ciudad de México. Newspaper *Sin Embargo*. Retrieved from www.sinembargo.mx/17-09-2017/3309860.

André, S. (1999). *What Does a Woman Want?* New York: Other Press.

Anzieu, D. (1989). *The Skin Ego*. New Haven, CT: Yale University Press.

Aulagnier, P. (2001 [1975]). *The Violence of Interpretation: From Pictogram to Statement*, translated by Alan Sheridan. Hove: Brunner-Routledge.

Bick, E. (1968). The Experience of the Skin in Early Object-Relations. *Int. J. Psycho-Anal.*, 49: 484–486.

Bion, W.R. (1970). *Attention and Interpretation: A Scientific Approach to Insight in Psycho-Analysis and Groups*. London: Tavistock.

Braunstein, N. (2016). *El discurso del psicoanálisis*. México:Siglo XXI.

Breuer, J. and Freud, S. (1893). On The Psychical Mechanism of Hysterical Phenomena. *The Standard Edition of the Complete Psychological Works of Sigmund Freud, Volume II (1893–1895): Studies on Hysteria*.

Butler, J. (1993). *Bodies that Matter: On the Discursive Limits of "Sex"*. New York: Routledge.

Butler, J. (1997). *Excitable Speech: A Politics of the Performative*. New York: Routledge.

Butler, J. (2000). *Antigone's Claim: Kinship between Life and Death*. New York: Columbia University Press.

Butler, J. (2016). Kinship Trouble in The Bacchae. Housman Lecture 2017. (2017). Retrieved from https://www.youtube.com/watch?v=ixwrw0PMC8I.

Capellá, A. (1996). *Lo histérico y lo obsesivo*. Barcelona: Herder.

Chemama, R. and Vanermersch, B. (1998). *Diccionario de Psicoanálisis*. Buenos Aires: Amorrortu.

Comisión Nacional para prevenir y erradicar la violencia contra las mujeres. (2016). Estadísticas sobre las modalidades de violencia contra las mujeres. México, gob.mx, April 6,

2016. Retrieved from https://www.gob.mx/conavim/articulos/conoce-algunas-estadisticas-sobre-las-modalidades-de-la-violencia-contra-las-mujeres?idiom=es.
David-Ménard, M. (1989). *Hysteria from Freud to Lacan: Body and Language in Psychoanalysis.* Ithaca, NY: Cornell University Press.
Derrida, J. and Dufourmantelle, A. (2000). *Of Hospitality.* Stanford, CA: Stanford University Press.
Didi-Hubermann, G. (2004). *Invention of Hysteria: Charcot and the Photographic Iconography of the Salpêtrière.* Cambridge, MA: The MIT Press.
Desarrollo Humano Y Violencia Contra Las Mujeres En México. (2016). México: Programa De Las Naciones Unidas Para El Desarrollo; Entidad De Las Naciones Unidas Para La Igualdad De Género Y El Empoderamiento De Las Mujeres. Instituto Nacional De Las Mujeres (INMUJERES, México), 2016. Retrieved from http://mexico.unwomen.org/es/digiteca/publicaciones/2016/01/desarrollo-humano-violencia-mujeres.
Dolto, F. (1984). *L'image inconsciente du corps.* Paris: Éditions du Seuil.
Freud, S. (1873). Letter from Sigmund Freud to Emil Fluss, March 17, 1873. *Letters of Sigmund Freud 1873–1939*, 1–2.
Freud, S. (1873). Letter from Sigmund Freud to Emil Fluss, June 16, 1873. *Letters of Sigmund Freud 1873–1939*, 3–6.
Freud, S. (1893). Letter dated November 27 1893, from Extracts from the Fliess Papers. *The Standard Edition of the Complete Psychological Works of Sigmund Freud.* Translated by James Strachey, in collaboration with Anna Freud and assisted by Alix Strachey and Alan Tyson. London: The Hogarth Press and The Institute of Psychoanalysis [Hereafter *CPWSF*]. *Volume I (1886–1899): Pre-Psycho-Analytic Publications and Unpublished Drafts*, 184–186.
Freud, S. (1893). Draft B. The Etiology of the Neuroses, February 8, 1893. *The Complete Letters of Sigmund Freud to Wilhelm Fliess, 1887–1904.*
Freud, S. (1893). The Psychotherapy of Hysteria from Studies on Hysteria. *CPWSF, Volume II (1893–1895): Studies on Hysteria.*
Freud, S. (1894). Draft G. Melancholia. *The Complete Letters of Sigmund Freud to Wilhelm Fliess, 1887–1904.*
Freud, S. (1895). Project for a Scientific Psychology. *CPWSF, Volume I (1886–1899): Pre-Psycho-Analytic Publications and Unpublished Drafts.*
Freud, S. (1896). Letter 52 from Extracts from the Fliess Papers. *CPWSF, Volume I (1886–1899): Pre-Psycho-Analytic Publications and Unpublished Drafts*, 233–239.
Freud, S. (1896). Further Remarks on the Neuro-Psychoses of Defence. *CPWSF, Volume III (1893–1899): Early Psycho-Analytic Publications.*
Freud, S. (1897). Freud to Fliess, Letter 69, September 21, 1897. Extracts from the Fliess Papers, 259–260; also in *Complete Letters of Freud to Fliess.*
Freud, S. (1897). Letter from Freud to Fliess, October 15, 1897. *The Complete Letters of Sigmund Freud to Wilhelm Fliess, 1887–1904*, 257–258.
Freud, S. (1897). Letter 71, Extracts from the Fliess Papers. *CPWSF, Volume I (1886–1899): Pre-Psycho-Analytic Publications and Unpublished Drafts*, 263–266.
Freud, S. (1897). Draft L, May 2, 1897. *The Complete Letters of Sigmund Freud to Wilhelm Fliess, 1887–1904*, 240–242.
Freud, S. (1899). Letter dated August 31, 1899 from Extracts from the Fliess Papers. *CPWSF, Volume I: Pre-Psycho-Analytic Publications and Unpublished Drafts*, 184–186.
Freud, S. (1899). Screen Memories. *CPWSF, Volume III (1893–1899): Early Psycho-Analytic Publications.*
Freud, S. (1900). The Interpretation of Dreams. *CPWSF, Volume IV (1900): The Interpretation of Dreams (First Part).*
Freud, S. (1905). Three Essays on the Theory of Sexuality. *CPWSF, Volume VII (1901–1905): A Case of Hysteria, Three Essays on Sexuality and Other Works.*

Freud, S. (1908). On the Sexual Theories of Children. *CPWSF, Volume IX (1906–1908): Jensen's "Gradiva" and Other Works.*
Freud, S. (1909). Analysis of a Phobia in a Five-Year-Old Boy. *CPWSF, Volume X (1909): Two Case Histories ("Little Hans" and the "Rat Man")*, 1–150.
Freud, S. (1909). Notes upon a Case of Obsessional Neurosis. *CPWSF, Volume X (1909): Two Case Histories ("Little Hans" and the "Rat Man")*, 151–318.
Freud, S. (1910). The Psycho-Analytic View of Psychogenic Disturbance of Vision. *CPWSF, Volume XI (1910): Five Lectures on Psycho-Analysis, Leonardo da Vinci and Other Works.*
Freud, S. (1910). A Special Type of Choice of Object made by Men (Contributions to the Psychology of Love I). *CPWSF, Volume XI (1910): Five Lectures on Psycho-Analysis, Leonardo da Vinci and Other Works*, 163–176.
Freud, S. (1913). Totem and Taboo. *CPWSF, Volume XIII (1913–1914): Totem and Taboo and Other Works.*
Freud, S. (1914). On Narcissism. *CPWSF, Volume XIV (1914–1916): On the History of the Psycho-Analytic Movement, Papers on Metapsychology and Other Works.*
Freud, S. (1915). Instincts and their Vicissitudes. *CPWSF, Volume XIV: On the History of the Psycho-Analytic Movement, Papers on Metapsychology and Other Works.*
Freud, S. (1915). The Unconscious. *CPWSF, Volume XIV (1914–1916): On the History of the Psycho-Analytic Movement, Papers on Metapsychology and Other Works.*
Freud, S. (1917). A Childhood Recollection from *Dichtung Und Wahrheit. CPWSF, Volume XVII (1917–1919): An Infantile Neurosis and Other Works*, 145–156.
Freud, S. (1918). From the History of an Infantile Neurosis. *CPWSF, Volume XVII (1917–1919): An Infantile Neurosis and Other Works*, 1–124.
Freud, S. (1920). Beyond the Pleasure Principle. *CPWSF, Volume XVIII (1920–1922): Beyond the Pleasure Principle, Group Psychology and Other Works.*
Freud, S. (1923). The Ego and the Id. *CPWSF, Volume XIX (1923–1925): The Ego and the Id and Other Works.*
Freud, S. (1923). The Infantile Genital Organization (An Interpolation into the Theory of Sexuality). *CPWSF, Volume XIX (1923–1925): The Ego and the Id and Other Works.*
Freud, S. (1924). The Dissolution of the Oedipus Complex. *CPWSF, Volume XIX (1923–1925): The Ego and the Id and Other Works.*
Freud, S. (1924). The Economic Problem of Masochism. *CPWSF, Volume XIX (1923–1925): The Ego and the Id and Other Works.*
Freud, S. (1925). A Note upon the "Mystic Writing-Pad". *CPWSF, Volume XIX (1923–1925): The Ego and the Id and Other Works*, 225–232.
Freud, S. (1925). Negation. *CPWSF, Volume XIX (1923–1925): The Ego and the Id and Other Works*, 233–240.
Freud, S. (1925). Some Psychical Consequences of the Anatomical Distinction between the Sexes. *CPWSF, Volume XIX (1923–1925): The Ego and the Id and Other Works*, 241–258.
Freud, S. (1928). Dostoevsky and Parricide. *CPWSF, Volume XXI (1927–1931): The Future of an Illusion, Civilization and its Discontents, and Other Works.*
Freud, S. (1930). Civilization and its Discontents. *CPWSF, Volume XXI (1927–1931): The Future of an Illusion, Civilization and its Discontents, and Other Works.*
Freud, S. (1931). Female Sexuality. *CPWSF, Volume XXI (1927–1931): The Future of an Illusion, Civilization and its Discontents, and Other Works*, 221–244.
Freud, S. (1933). *CPWSF, Volume XXII: New Introductory Lectures on Psychoanalysis.*
Freud, S. (1937). Analysis Terminable and Interminable. *CPWSF, Volume XXIII (1937–1939): Moses and Monotheism: An Outline of Psycho-Analysis and Other Works.*
Freud, S. (1938). An Outline of Psycho-Analysis. *CPWSF, Volume XXIII (1937–1939): Moses and Monotheism: An Outline of Psycho-Analysis and Other Works.*

Freud, S. (1938). Findings, Ideas, Problems. *CPWSF, Volume XXIII (1937–1939): Moses and Monotheism: An Outline of Psycho-Analysis and Other Works.*

Green, A. (2011). *The Tragic Effect: The Oedipus Complex in Tragedy*. Cambridge, MA: Harvard University Press.

Jones, E. (1954). *The Life and Work of Sigmund Freud*. London: The Hogarth Press.

Khomami, N. (2017). #MeToo: How a hashtag became a rallying cry against sexual harassment. *The Guardian*, October 20, 2017. Retrieved from https://www.theguardian.com/world/2017/oct/20/women-worldwide-use-hashtag-metoo-against-sexual-harassment.

Kristeva, J. (1982). *Powers of Horror: An Essay on Abjection*. New York: Columbia University Press.

Lacan, J. (1958). *The Formations of the Unconscious*. The Seminars of Jacques Lacan. Book V. New York: Norton.

Lacan, J. (1959–1960). *The Ethics of Psychoanalysis*. The Seminars of Jacques Lacan. Book VII. New York: Norton.

Lacan, J. (1972). *Encore. On Feminine Sexuality: The Limits of Love and Knowledge*. The Seminars of Jacques Lacan. Book XX. New York: Norton.

Laplanche, J. (1984). La pulsion et son objet-source. Son destin et le transfert. *Annuel de l'APF*, 2014(1): 201–216.

Laplanche, J. (1985). *Life and Death in Psychoanalysis*. Baltimore, MD: Johns Hopkins University Press.

Laplanche, J. (1997). The Theory of Seduction and the Problem of the Other. *Int. J. Psycho-Anal.*, 78: 653–666.

Laplanche, J. and Pontalis, J.B. (1968). Fantasy and the Origins of Sexuality 1. *Int. J. Psycho-Anal.*, 49: 1–18.

Laplanche, J. and Pontalis, J. B. (1998). *The Language of Psychoanalysis*. London: Karnac Books.

McDougall, J. (1989). *Theaters of the Body: A Psychoanalytic Approach to Psychosomatic Illness*. New York: Norton.

McDougall, J. (1993). *Plea for a Measure of Abnormality*. London: Routledge.

Postel, J. and Quetel, J. (1983). *Nueva historia de la psiquiatría*. México: Fondo de Cultura Económico.

Preciado, P.B. (2012). Somatheque. Producción biopolítica, feminismos, prácticas queer y trans. Conference. Retrieved from www.museoreinasofia.es/actividades/somateca-presentacion-programa-practicas-criticas.

Preciado, P.B. (2013) *Testo Junkie: Sex, Drugs and Politics in the Pharmacopornographic Era*. New York: The Feminist Press.

Preciado, P.B. (2014). July 10. Inappropriate Bodies. Conference at Museo de Arte Contemporáneo Barcelona. Podcast. Retrieved from www.macba.cat/es/audio-beatriz-preciado-cuerpos-inapropiables.

Prengler, A. (2001). El niño del carretel: una visita a W. Ernest Freud. Revista Fort-Da No. 3. Retrieved from www.fort-da.org/fort-da3/ernest.htm.

Roudinesco, É. (2006). *La Familia en desorden*. México: Fondo de Cultura Económica.

Roudinesco, É. (2015). Por qué el psicoanálisis se debe renovar. Newspaper *El País*, September 4. Retrieved from http://cultura.elpais.com/cultura/2015/09/02/babelia/1441210297_491115.html.

Roudinesco, É. (2016). *Freud: In His Time and Ours*. Cambridge, MA: Harvard University Press.

Schwab, G.B. (1838). *Sagen des klassischen Altertums* [Legends of classical antiquity]. Frankfurt: Insel Verlag.

Sophocles. (2003). *Theban Plays*, edited by P. Meineck and P. Woodruff. Indianapolis, IN: Hackett.

Sophocles. (1958). *The Oedipus Plays of Sophocles: Oedipus the King, Oedipus at Colonus, Antigone*, edited by P. Roche. New York: New American Library.

Treszesamsky, J. (2015). Edipo en la biblioteca de Freud. Retrieved from https://historiasdelpsicoanalisis.wordpress.com/2015/01/19/edipo-en-la-biblioteca-de-freud/.

Valencia, A. (2002). Transferencia y Acción Específica. Carta Psi. Retrieved from www.cartapsi.org/new/transferencia-y-accion-especifica/.

Valencia, A. (2017). El Objeto del Psicoanálisis o lo Que Acontece en el Cuerpo. Carta Psi. Article. Retrieved from www.cartapsi.org/new/el-objeto-del-psicoanalisis-o-lo-que-acontece-en-el-cuerpo/.

Wolheim, R. and Hopkins, J. (1982). *Philosophical Essays on Freud: The Bodily Ego*. Cambridge: Cambridge University Press, 124–138.

INDEX

For Product Safety Concerns and Information please contact our EU representative GPSR@taylorandfrancis.com
Taylor & Francis Verlag GmbH, Kaufingerstraße 24, 80331 München, Germany

www.ingramcontent.com/pod-product-compliance
Ingram Content Group UK Ltd.
Pitfield, Milton Keynes, MK11 3LW, UK
UKHW022314250926
475702UK00046B/776

9781138388420